Carl Wood and Alan Trounson

Clinical In Vitro Fertilization

Second Edition

With 20 Figures

Springer-Verlag
London Berlin Heidelberg New York
Paris Tokyo

Carl Wood, CBE, FRCS, FRCOG, FRACOG
Chairman, Department of Obstetrics and Gynaecology, Monash
University, Monash Medical Centre, Clayton, Victoria, Australia

Alan Trounson, MSc, PhD
Director, Centre for Early Human Development, Monash
University, Monash Medical Centre, Clayton, Victoria, Australia

Front cover: SEM of "non-receptive" uterus showing long regular microvilli.

ISBN-13: 978-1-4471-1666-0   e-ISBN-13: 978-1-4471-1664-6
DOI: 10.1007/ 978-1-4471-1664-6

British Library Cataloguing in Publication Data
Clinical in vitro fertilization.—2nd ed.
1. Women. Ova. In vitro fertilization
I. Wood, Carl, *1929* II. Trounson, Alan, *1946* 612'.62

Library of Congress Cataloguing-in-Publication Data
Clinical in vitro fertilization.
Includes bibliographies and index. 1. Fertilization in vitro, Human. I. Wood, Carl.
II. Trounson, Alan. [DNLM: 1. Embryo Transfer. 2. Fertilization In Vitro.
WQ 205 C6405] RG135.C57 1988   618.1'78059   88-24847

© Springer-Verlag Berlin Heidelberg 1989
Softcover reprint of the hardcover 1st edition 1989
The use of registered names, trademarks, etc. in this publication does not imply,
even in the absence of a specific statement, that such names are exempt from the
relevant laws and regulations and therefore free for general use.

Product Liability: The publisher can give no guarantee for information about drug
dosage and application thereof contained in this book. In every individual case the
respective user must check its accuracy by consulting other pharmaceutical literature.

Typeset by Wilmaset, Birkenhead, Merseyside

2128/3916-543210 (Printed on acid-free paper)

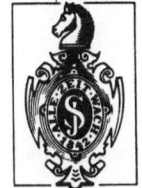

Preface to the Second Edition

In vitro fertilization has resulted in an estimated 4000–5000 births in the world. The procedure has been accepted in Europe, America and Australia and several hundred IVF clinics are operating successfully.

The newer procedures of GIFT, embryo freezing and donor oocyte IVF have become established and are dealt with in several chapters. GIFT has become the procedure of choice for patients with infertility of unknown origin. Oocyte freezing represents an important new technology which is being developed. The routine IVF procedure has improved slightly; variation in results can be reduced by quality control of laboratory and clinical techniques. Male factor infertility has been dealt with by IVF in mild and moderate cases, but newer techniques will be required to deal with severe problems in the male.

Most countries have accepted that the straightforward IVF procedure is ethical. Limitations concerning the use of donor oocytes and embryo experimentation exist in some religions and countries; legal control of the new reproductive technologies ranges from the passage of statutes to no control at all. Many countries are still considering the need for legislative control.

The text endeavours to indicate new areas of importance and to guide those organizing services as to how to introduce newer technologies.

Melbourne, 1988   Carl Wood, Alan Trounson

Preface to the First Edition

Man is entering a new era as a result of advances in human reproduction. Techniques have been developed to assist in the creation of man—artificial insemination and, now, in vitro fertilization (IVF). Soon, other new methods, based upon current advances of the IVF procedure, will develop to improve the quality of human reproduction. The book describes the conceptual framework and details of technique concerned with in vitro fertilization and embryo transfer (ET).

Edwards and Steptoe first described the technique of IVF and ET and the subsequent births of two normal babies. Since then, the success rate of the system has been improved by the use of fertility drugs to provide more oocytes and preincubation to mature the oocyte before fertilization. As a result of the continued research from Melbourne and Cambridge, more than 100 babies have been born.

A free interchange of information between the Cambridge and Melbourne groups has led to a predictable success rate of 15%–20% per laparoscopy, and infertility centres all over the world are now copying the techniques. It is an appropriate time to inform doctors and scientists to help them understand the various procedures involved in IVF and ET. While many advances will occur in the future, the establishment of high success rates in several of the critical steps in the procedure—oocyte pick-up rate (90%), fertilization (>90%) and early embryo development (70%–90%)—signifies that some of the new techniques are stabilized sufficiently to warrant transmission of information by text, rather than scientific journal.

In vitro fertilization and embryo transfer is now a practical method of treating certain types of infertility. Its development has far greater implications. Hitherto, medicine has been restricted to preventing and treating disease. It is now possible to assist in man's creation. This has social and ethical consequences which require serious consideration by the community, as well as by the medical profession. The increased knowledge of human reproduction resulting from the development of the technique of IVF and ET will assist in the development of new contraceptives and in understanding the causes of certain fetal malformations.

This book endeavours to inform the medical profession of the current scientific status of IVF and ET, the history and future of the technique and the ethical, psychological and social consequences of their development.

Melbourne, 1983   Carl Wood, Alan Trounson

Contents

Contributors

Louise Bowen, Dip. Soc. Stud. Infertility Counselling Co-ordinator, Infertility Medical Centre, Melbourne, Victoria, Australia.

I. T. Cameron, MD, MRCOG, MRACOG. Senior Registrar Royal Women's Hospital, Melbourne, Victoria, Australia.

C. Chen, AM, FRCOG, FRACOG, FICS, FACS. Head, Department of Obstetrics and Gynaecology 'B' Unit; Director, IVF and Gamete Research Centre; Director, National Sperm Bank, Kandang Kerbau Hospital, Hampshire Road, Singapore, Republic of Singapore.

D. M. de Kretser, MMBS, MD. Professor of Anatomy, Monash University, Melbourne; Co-Director, Reproductive Medicine Clinic, Prince Henry's Hospital, Melbourne, Victoria, Australia.

D. L. Healy, MBBS (Hons), PhD, FRACOG. Wellcome Trust Senior Clinical Research Fellow, Medical Research Centre, Prince Henry's Hospital, Melbourne, Victoria, Australia; Honorary Senior Lecturer, Monash University, Department of Obstetrics & Gynaecology, Monash Medical Centre, Melbourne, Victoria, Australia and Chairman, Subdivision of Reproductive Medicine, Monash Medical Centre, Melbourne, Victoria, Australia.

R. P. S. Jansen, MBBS, MD, BMedSci, FRACP, MRCOG, FRACOG, MAFS. Director of Fertility Services, Royal Prince Alfred's Hospital, Sydney; Chairman Sydney IVF, Sydney, NSW, Australia.

H. W. Jones Jr, MD. Reproductive Medicine, Department of Obstetrics and Gynaecology, Eastern Virginia Medical School, Norfolk, Virginia, 23507 USA.

G. T. Kovacs, MBBS (Hons), FRACOG, FRCOG. Clinical Director, Monash/Epworth IVF Programme, Senior Lecturer, Department of Obstetrics and Gynaecology, Monash Medical Centre, Melbourne, Victoria, Australia.

P. A. L. Lancaster, MBBS, MPH, FRACP. Director, National Perinatal Statistics Unit, University of Sydney, New South Wales, Australia.

J. Leeton, FRACS, MGO, FRCOG, FRACOG. Associate Professor, Monash University, Department of Obstetrics and Gynaecology, Monash Medical Centre, Melbourne, Victoria, Australia.

P. Lutjen, PhD. Senior Scientific Officer, Department of O & G, Royal North Shore Hospital, Sydney, NSW, Australia.

C. Murphy, PhD. Senior Lecturer, Department of Histology and Embryology, University of Sydney, NSW, Australia.

Kay Oke, Dip. Soc. Stud. Infertility Counsellor, Royal Women's Hospital, Melbourne, Victoria, Australia.

P. A. W. Rogers, PhD. Senior Research Fellow, Monash University, Department of Obstetrics and Gynaecology, Monash Medical Centre, Melbourne, Victoria, Australia.

Caroline Thomas, BSc (Hons). Embryologist, Infertility Medical Centre, Epworth, Melbourne, Victoria, Australia.

A. Trounson, MSc, PhD. Reader, Department of Obstetrics and Gynaecology; Director, Centre for Early Human Development, Monash University, Monash Medical Centre, Melbourne, Victoria, Australia.

C. Wood, CBE, FRCS, FRCOG, FRACOG. Chairman, Monash University, Department of Obstetrics and Gynaecology, Monash Medical Centre, Melbourne, Victoria, Australia.

C. A. Yates, BSc (Hons). Chief Scientist of Andrology, Infertility Centre, Epworth, Melbourne, Victoria, Australia.

1 Selection and Preparation of Patients for In Vitro Fertilization

G. T. Kovacs

1.1 Introduction

When the use of in vitro fertilization (IVF) and embryo transfer (ET) first eventuated it was to bypass the fallopian tubes (Steptoe and Edwards 1979). When the first edition of *Clinical in vitro fertilization* was published in 1984 (Wood and Trounson 1984) it was already suggested that the technique may have wider applications. The prediction that "there will be rapid progress in the future" has been proved correct, and areas that were discussed as "future prospects" are now accepted clinical treatments. Its application to unexplained infertility was shown in 1983 (Mahadevan et al. 1983), and its use in the management of male infertility is now well established (de Kretser et al. 1985). Further applications of techniques for in vitro fertilization include the transfer of donated eggs and embryos (Trounson et al. 1983). With all these developments in vitro fertilization has been looked upon as the panacea for all causes of infertility. Current indications for the clinical use of in vitro fertilization in 1987 are listed in Table 1.1.

In Australia in vitro fertilization units have been established in all major cities, several having more than one unit. As IVF has been incorporated into the clinical treatment of all areas of subfertility therapy, specialist centres for subfertility/reproductive biology cannot function properly without an IVF unit. In the Monash University–Epworth Hospital–Queen Victoria Medical Centre unit there are more than 6000 patients on the waiting list. It is important that the management and preparation of these patients is organized in an orderly fashion. To enable this an efficient waiting list must be established.

1.2 The Waiting List

All relevant information, both of an epidemiological and a scientific nature, for each couple is recorded on a standardized form. Such a form should be computer

Table 1.1.   Indications for in vitro fertilization 1988

Tubal disease
Tubal disease not suitable for surgery
Unsuccessful surgery
Patent but abnormal tubes
Unexplained infertility
Endometriosis – completed therapy
Male subfertility
Oligospermia
Low motility
Abnormal morphology
Antisperm antibodies
Failed donor insemination
Cervical hostility
Failed ovulation induction
Absent or inappropriate oocytes
Absent/abnormal ovaries
Premature menopause
Genetic disease
Therapy for female cancer – embryo freezing prior to chemotherapy/cytotoxics
Absent uterus
Partial surrogacy

compatible and sufficient detail should be included so that specific clinical situations may be identified; for example, if a special research project is to be undertaken on patients who have had endometriosis, and this information is not recorded on the waiting list form, then it would be necessary to refer to all clinical notes to select appropriate patients. A controversial area is the allocation of priorities within the waiting list. It is our policy to allocate patients strictly chronologically and only allow patients to jump the waiting list on the basis of medical indications as judged by two members of the team. Other units have the policy of allocated priorities by taking into consideration such factors as previous children, the age of the couple and other social factors.

Special subgroups of research interest may need to jump the waiting list at times so that improvements from research may be incorporated as quickly as possible into the routine procedure. Our unit has a policy of having a throughput of up to 10% of couples in the "research category". Although the state Government in Victoria has established a special committee to study inclusion criteria and selection procedures, no firm recommendations have resulted. It is no longer our policy to put women who are 39 years or older on the waiting list, and to limit those already on the waiting list who are past the age of 40 to a maximum of three cycles of treatment.

1.2.1   Patient Activation

Just prior to commencing treatment the couple are interviewed by their Specialist Gynaecologist and any change in their medical condition is noted. The procedure of in vitro fertilization is again explained and the preliminary tests (as described below) are collated. Once patients have been activated they are eligible to enter treatment cycles.

1.3   Length of Menstrual Cycles – Confidence Limits

From the time of enrolment of couples on to the IVF waiting list the female partners are requested to maintain a menstrual calendar showing the first day of menstruation. From this record the length of their menstrual cycles, and subsequently the confidence limits for estimated ovulation, are calculated (McIntosh et al. 1980). The confidence limits are used to calculate when stimulation should begin, and when 8-hourly assays for luteinizing hormone (LH) should be commenced.

1.4   Hormonal Assessment

All patients have midluteal assessment of oestradiol (E_2), progesterone (P_4), follicle stimulating hormone (FSH), luteinizing hormone (LH) and prolactin. This confirms spontaneous ovulation, detects hyperprolactinaemia and also occult polycystic ovarian disease. If significant hyperprolactinaemia is detected it is important to exclude pituitary lesions and thyroid dysfunction before embarking on a pregnancy. Elevated prolactin levels are normalized using bromocryptine before IVF treatment commences. Patients with occult polycystic ovarian disease as shown by an excess of LH to FSH may need different stimulation, FSH or buserelin.

1.5   Assessment of Semen

All couples undergoing in vitro fertilization have a current semen analysis performed by a laboratory experienced in such work before entering a treatment cycle. In order to predict semen problems we recommend that two analyses should have been undertaken during the previous six months. Analysis of the semen sample should include assessment of volume, count, concentration, motility, motility index, morphology distribution, the number of inflammatory cells, the percentage of live cells and whether it was a total specimen.

1.5.1   Provision of Semen

Another advantage of the preliminary semen analyses is that if the male partner has problems with masturbation this will be identified early. The female partner is sometimes involved in helping to produce a specimen. In order to minimize the problem of inability to produce semen under stress a quiet private room is provided for the husband to masturbate, both in the pre-treatment work-up and also during the treatment cycle. This room has a selection of "Girly magazines" which some husbands find helpful. We have not resorted to the use of blue movies or telephone arousal services which have been suggested by some workers. Occasionally, if the husband has ongoing difficulty with masturbation, "back-up" semen can be frozen and stored for use if a fresh specimen cannot be produced. The use of special non-toxic condoms such as the Semen Collection Device (Neurotech) is available for couples where the husband has difficulty with masturbation.

1.5.2 Preliminary Sperm-wash Preparation

In men whose sperm concentration and/or motility is borderline we have instituted the routine of undertaking a preliminary "sperm-wash" procedure. In this situation the routine sperm preparation as used for in vitro fertilization is carried out. The initial sperm concentration and motility, as well as the final motility and the number of motile sperm recovered, is recorded. It is then calculated how many eggs it would be possible to inseminate with these recovered spermatazoa; this is then used as a guide to couples who are about to enter the programme for the treatment of a male factor.

1.5.3 Immunological Studies

All seminal plasma samples are tested with immunobeads for the presence of IgG and IgA antibodies. If antibodies are present a split ejaculate collection is used. As the presence of anti-sperm antibodies in the serum of the female partner is an occasional cause for failure of fertilization, we have introduced routine screening of female partners for anti-sperm antibodies prior to IVF therapy.

1.5.4 Microbiological Assessment of Semen

It used to be the practice of the Monash unit to perform several bacterial cultures on semen specimens before and during IVF. Now we only culture semen during the treatment cycle to exclude pathogens being introduced into the culture system. In pre-treatment semen analysis we find the presence of leucocytes a better index of infection. As infection can interfere with fertilization, and often no organisms are cultured, it is our practice to treat men who have more than six leucocytes per high power field with a course of erythromycin or doxycycline prior to IVF.

1.6 Serological Assessment

1.6.1 Female Partner

Serological assessment of the female partner is undertaken for rubella, hepatitis B, and HIV III. Although in the past we used to screen for toxoplasma, syphilis, cytomegalo virus and chlamydia, these tests have now been abandoned as they are of little value in preventing problems. The retrospective analysis of chlamydia antibodies showed a significantly increased incidence in women with tubal as opposed to idiopathic infertility (Asche et al. 1986), but was of no value in predicting current infection. Single estimates of plasma levels of toxoplasma or cytomegalo virus are also of little help in predicting current infection and therefore have been abandoned. Tests for syphilis have also been abandoned; it is probably more sensible to carry out screening during early pregnancy, as treatment of isolated cases antenatally will prevent congenital infection.

1.6.1.1 Rubella

Rubella immunity is assessed by haemagglutination inhibition titre. It is imperative that before patients embark on such a complicated therapy, the risk of rubella infection in pregnancy be prevented. Patients who are not immune are immunized and are asked to wait for three months before proceeding to attempt in vitro fertilization.

1.6.1.2 Hepatitis B Antigens

Testing for hepatitis is important in order to safeguard the staff as well as to diagnose any possible infection. All patients have numerous blood tests and maternal serum is used in the preparation of culture medium, so if an infected patient was not screened it could affect the culture system as well as possibly infecting the staff.

1.6.1.3 Human Immunodeficiency Virus (HIV)

Testing for HIV was commenced in 1985. There were several reasons for this. Although IVF patients are at low risk for carrying the virus, there is an anxiety among the staff about being infected that is out of all proportion to the risk of catching this disease. Secondly, if embryos are to be stored, or if eggs or embryos are donated, it is imperative to exclude the presence of HIV. Thirdly, should any patient subsequently have a positive test after treatment, it would be important to document whether the infection was already present prior to entering the programme or whether infection occurred as a result of treatment.

1.6.2 Male Partner

All male partners undergo a blood test for HIV III titre as well. As the semen has to be handled in the laboratory during the preparation of the spermatozoa, it is important to exclude the presence of the HIV. There are also medico-legal implications for the female partner.

1.7 Bacteriological Assessment of the Cervix

The routine of carrying out cervical bacteriology prior to each treatment cycle has now been abandoned. Should patients have abnormal symptoms or excessive discharge then cervical cultures would be undertaken. We undertook the routine examination of cervical secretions (culture and immunofluorescence) of the cervix for the presence of chlamydia, but our pickup rate was too low to justify routine screening.

It has now been shown that the risk factors for chlamydia include multiple sexual partners (Kovacs et al. 1988), and couples undergoing in vitro fertilization are not usually in this category.

1.8   Assessment of the Pelvis Prior to Treatment

In order to properly assess the female partner preliminary laparoscopy prior to IVF is mandatory. This assessment should have been carried out within a year or two of entering the programme. At this examination the accessibility of the ovaries and the normality of the tubes should be assessed. With recent evidence suggesting that gamete intra-fallopian transfer (GIFT) has significantly higher pregnancy rates in cases of idiopathic infertility than routine IVF and ET (Molloy et al. 1987) the decision to proceed in this direction will have to be made after laparoscopy. It is also important that other complicating factors such as endometriosis are excluded. If the unit is using only laparoscopic oocyte collection then the accessibility of the ovaries has to be assessed carefully. With the use of hyperstimulation and the development of multiple follicles, some access to both or one ovary is still necessary. It has to be kept in mind that the eventual outcome of IVF and ET is related to the number of mature oocytes collected; the better the access the greater the chance of success.

With the change towards vaginal ultrasonic oocyte retrieval, and harvest rates for this technique similar to those of laparoscopy (Kovacs et al. 1988), laparoscopic accessibility of the ovaries has become less important. Some of the manoeuvres which were previously undertaken to improve laparoscopic access are a handicap for trans-vaginal ultrasonic retrieval. The habit of suturing ovaries to the uterine fundus, although enhancing the laparoscopic pickup, is a grave disadvantage for vaginal access. If access is not possible either by laparoscopy or by vaginal ultrasound, the use of transvesical abdominal ultrasonic follicular puncture may need to be employed (Lenz 1985). Careful assessment prior to entering the programme will enable appropriate preparations to be made for a suitable route for oocyte retrieval.

1.9   Consent Forms

With the various computations and permutations available for in vitro fertilization, consent forms need to cover the following areas: the technique of in vitro fertilization, its potential complications, the inability to guarantee success and possible unknown ill effects on the resultant fetus. Should the use of donor sperm or eggs be contemplated then the appropriate consent form would have to be signed. Similarly if the couple may donate excess eggs and/or embryos they will also have to consent to this. If excess embryos or eggs are to be frozen special consent is obtained outlining the experimental nature of these procedures. Despite the presence of signed consent forms suggesting all care but no responsibility, they do not absolve the team from responsibility. Each member of the team is expected to act with the care and competence of a standard as practised by experts in the particular field. Should a misfortune result and action for negligence be taken, the onus is on the team to show that all reasonable care has been taken. The main reason for having consent forms is to provide written evidence that the couple have given consent and the consent was "informed", meaning that the couple who had the treatment had the possible complications explained and understood. As legal systems vary from state to state and country to country, it is advised that appropriate legal advice be obtained before the consent forms are drafted.

1.10　Psychological Preparation

Most couples entering the in vitro fertilization programme have been through a long series of investigations. They often are depressed about their inability to conceive and, not infrequently, one or other of the partners feels inadequate at not being able to fulfil the spouse's desire for a child. Sometimes there is pressure from one or the other partner that if the child is not produced then divorce may result. Some women feel resentful about other couples with young children and feel particularly aggressive against women having pregnancies terminated. Loss of libido is not uncommon. Many couples find that intercourse becomes a calculated compulsory activity and all element of pleasure and recreation is removed. Some men become impotent and unable to perform. If couples understand the natural grief reaction which their loss of fertility produces, that is denial, depression, anxiety, anger and resentment, then it will be easier to cope with these emotional states. Many couples find they can cope with these problems on their own, whereas others find the patient support group very helpful (see below). Some need to see a counsellor and a very small minority may require the help of a psychologist or psychiatrist.

It is also important that patients have adequate written information about infertility problems and in vitro fertilization. We have produced several relevant publications: an *Infertility patient handbook* (Kovacs and Wood 1984), a book specifically explaining in vitro fertilization *Test tube conception* (Wood and Westmore 1983), as well as a special instruction book on the *Monash University Infertility Medical Centre in vitro fertilization program* (Fig. 1.1). Some couples found that their emotional state improved while they were on the waiting list. When they have had no prospects of pregnancy previously, the thought that treatment is available may give them new hope.

We also encourage the exploring of other alternatives such as adoption, fostering and child-free existence. We feel that only if all possible avenues are explored, can couples make rational decisions about which option to pursue.

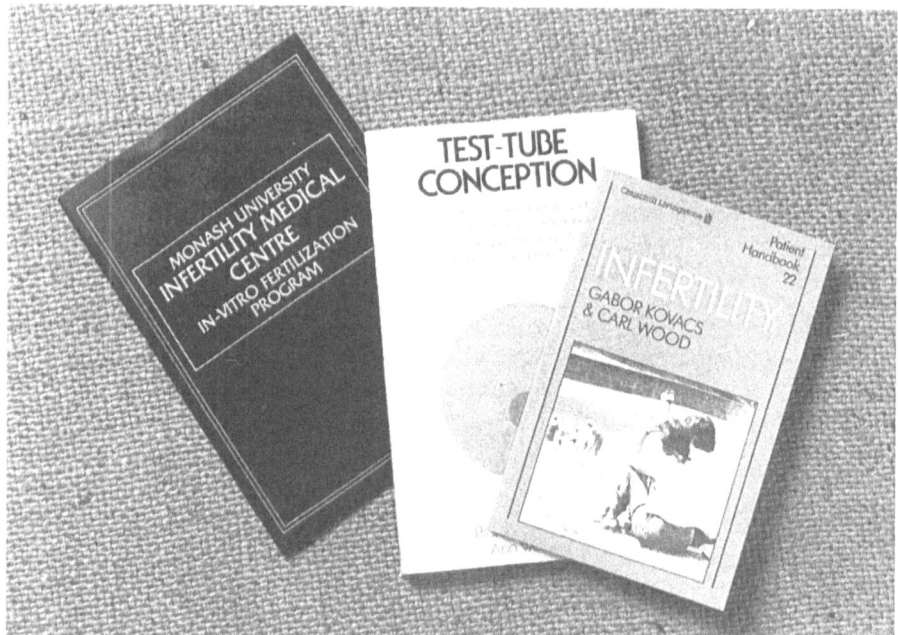

Fig. 1.1.   Books recommended to all patients on the IVF waiting list.

1.11   Patient Support Group

Since the very early days of IVF, a patient support group has been active. Its first aim was to raise funds to support the programme before it became financially viable. It then extended its activities to provide support to couples on the waiting list. Now the group has an important political role as it makes submissions to various government committees as well as giving feedback to the management committee of the IVF programme. The Monash IVF Friends produces a monthly newsletter and has regular meetings at which members of the IVF team are invited to make a presentation. This results in better communication between the team and consumers.

References

Asche V, King H, Kovacs GT, Westcott M (1986) *Chlamydia trachomatis* infection in 1300 fertile and infertile women in Melbourne. In: Proceedings of the XII world congress on fertility and sterility. Singapore, 26–31 October 1986, p 223

de Kretser DM, Yates C, Kovacs GT (1985) The use of IVF in the management of male infertility. Clin Obstet Gynaecol 12:767–773

Kovacs GT, Wood C (1984) Infertility. Churchill Livingstone, Edinburgh (Patient handbook 22)

Kovacs GT, Westcott M, Rusden J et al. (1988) The incidence of *Chlamydia trachomatis* in a young sexually active population. Med J Aust (in press)

Kovacs GT, King C, Cushanan L, Wood C (1988) The outcome of in vitro fertilization – the comparison of vaginal ultrasound and laparoscopic ovum retrieval. (in press)
Lenz S (1985) Percutaneous oocyte recovery using ultrasound. Clin Obstet Gynaecol 12:785–798
Mahadevan MM, Trounson AO, Leeton JF (1983) The relationship of tubal blockage, infertility of unknown cause, suspected male infertility and endometriosis to success of in vitro fertilization and embryo transfer. Fertil Steril 40:755–762
McIntosh JEA, Matthews CD, Crocker JM, Broom TJ, Coc LW (1980) Predicting the luteinizing hormone surge: relationship between the duration of the follicular and luteal phases and the length of the human menstrual cycle. Fertil Steril 34:125–130
Molloy D, Speirs A, duPlessis Y, McBain J, Johnston I (1987) A laparoscopic approach to a program of gamete intrafallopian transfer. Fertil Steril 47:289–293
Steptoe PC, Edwards RG (1979) Birth after the re-implantation of a human embryo. Lancet II:366
Trounson A, Leeton J, Besanko M, Wood C, Conti A (1983) Pregnancy established in an infertile patient after transfer of a donated embryo fertilized in vitro. Br Med J 286:835–838
Wood C, Trounson A (eds) (1984) Clinical in vitro fertilization. Springer-Verlag, Berlin Heidelberg New York

2 Patient Management

I. T. Cameron and D. L. Healy

2.1 Introduction

The successful in vitro fertilization (IVF) of a single oocyte from the dominant follicle in a natural ovarian cycle was classically demonstrated by the birth of· Louise Brown in 1978. However, the realization that IVF pregnancy rates could be improved with multiple embryo transfer led to the use of ovarian stimulation as a means of attaining multiple follicular development (Trounson et al. 1981). It is now usual to undertake ovarian stimulation in the IVF treatment cycle, often with combinations of clomiphene citrate (CC), human menopausal gonadotrophin (hMG), and human chorionic gonadotrophin (hCG) (Garcia et al. 1983; Jones et al. 1983; Laufer et al. 1983; Rogers et al. 1986).

This chapter will discuss theoretical and practical aspects of the stimulation regimen employed in the Monash University IVF programme. However, it is first appropriate to consider the physiological process of folliculogenesis leading to ovulation and luteinization in the natural cycle.

2.2 Natural Folliculogenesis

There are about 200 million primordial follicles in the human ovary at birth. Most of these are destined to become atretic and, in a fertile woman having regular monthly cycles for 35 years, only 400 or so ovulatory follicles would be expected to develop. The most dramatic changes in any particular follicle are seen in the 2 weeks prior to ovulation itself.

The human primordial follicle measures 0.05 mm in diameter (Baker 1963). On day 1 of the menstrual cycle, the antral follicle is 4 mm in size and contains 1 million granulosa cells, but by ovulation the follicle has grown to 20–25 mm and contains 50 million granulosa cells (McNatty et al. 1979). Understanding the endocrine mechanisms controlling this 50-fold growth has come from a number of studies in the rhesus monkey and the sheep (Hodgen 1982; Baird 1983; Goodman and Hodgen 1983).

The precursory primary follicle contains an oocyte surrounded by a single layer of spindle-shaped cells. Next, the primordial follicle contains one or more layers of recognizable granulosa cells, but no fluid-filled antrum is seen. On the other hand, a secondary follicle contains a variable volume of antral fluid which increases markedly as the graafian follicle approaches ovulation (Ross and van de Wiele, 1981). Follicle recruitment, which normally occurs during the first few days of the primate ovarian cycle, is the process whereby the follicle continues to mature in the correct gonadotrophic environment to allow progress towards ovulation. Recruited follicles correspond to small antral follicles. Selection is the mechanism by which a single follicle is chosen and ultimately the selected follicle alone can avoid atresia to achieve ovulation. Dominance is the method by which the selected follicle maintains its pre-eminence over all other follicles (Goodman et al. 1977) and occupies days 8–12 of the primate ovarian cycle, after which the corpus luteum reigns from about day 16 to day 24 (Fig. 2.1).

Only those follicles which have been exposed to the optimum sequence of follicle stimulating hormone (FSH) and luteinizing hormone (LH) will avoid atresia. In the luteal phase gonadotrophin levels are low due to oestradiol and progesterone negative feedback; at that stage all follicles greater than 4 mm are atretic (McNatty et al. 1983). Further follicular development can only occur following removal of the corpus luteum (Nilsson et al. 1982; Baird et al. 1984), or the administration of exogenous gonadotrophin (diZerega and Hodgen 1980); this suggests that although small antral follicle development requires low concentrations of FSH, larger amounts are necessary to promote subsequent growth. Such development may occur once a threshold level of FSH has been attained (Brown 1978) and a 20% increase in the concentration of FSH, as might occur in the early proliferative phase, is sufficient to stimulate follicular development beyond 4 mm. Granulosa aromatase activity results in high local concentrations of oestradiol in the selected follicle and dominance is achieved by inhibiting FSH secretion with oestradiol and inhibin (Baird and Fraser 1975; Findlay 1986). In addition, the secretion of a follicle regulatory protein by the dominant follicle may impair the sensitivity of other follicles to gonadotrophin stimulation (Ono et al. 1986).

Thus, although folliculogenesis is dependent on FSH and LH, the early stages are probably independent of cyclical gonadotrophin concentrations until the follicle reaches the small antral stage. Thereafter, further development will only occur in the face of an increase in FSH concentrations above the threshold level, allowing only those follicles at the appropriate stage of maturity to proceed. The interval during which FSH remains elevated above the threshold level can be seen as a gate through which a follicle must pass to avoid atresia on the path towards ovulation. The width of the gate will therefore determine the number of follicles that can be selected for ovulation (Baird 1987).

2.2.1 Luteinization and Ovulation

The pre-ovulatory LH surge is triggered by the positive feedback of oestradiol from the dominant follicle, and this action has been reproduced using exogenous

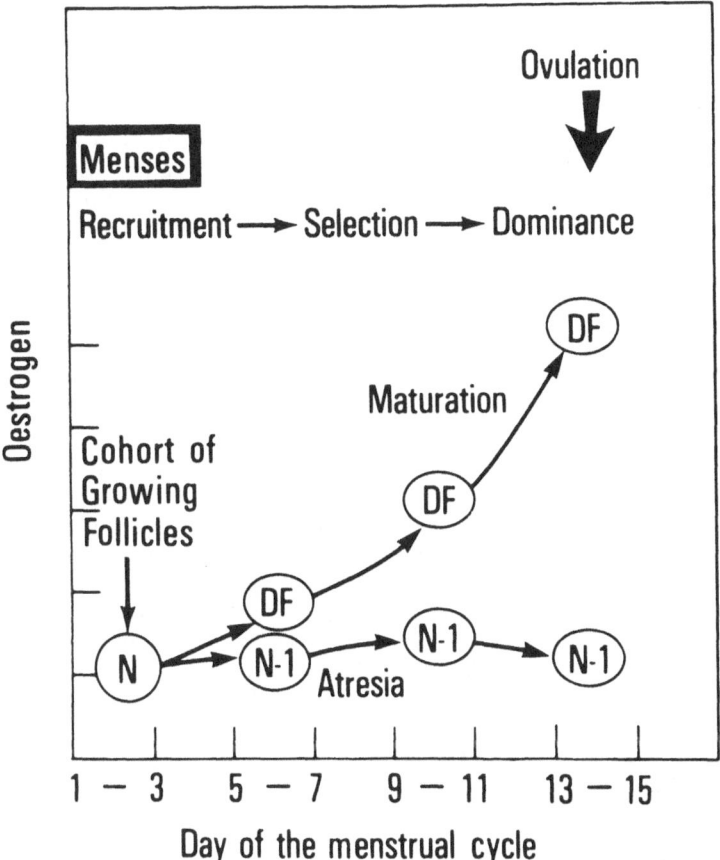

Fig. 2.1. Selection and maturation of the dominant follicle (DF). N, cohort of 4 mm antral follicles available for recruitment.

oestrogen in women (Nillius and Wide 1971). However, it is likely that other follicular factors also contribute to the LH triggering mechanism, for the LH surge can be initiated from widely differing serum oestradiol concentrations. The rate of change of oestrogen levels, and alterations in the synthesis of inhibitors such as inhibin, may also play a role.

In addition, a pre-ovulatory increase in progesterone may facilitate the LH surge in both monkeys (Schenken et al. 1985) and women (Odell and Swerdloff 1968; Leyendecker et al. 1976). Indeed, the administration of the progesterone receptor antagonist RU486 to *Cynomologus* monkeys delayed or blocked the mid-cycle gonadotrophin surge, resulting in atresia of the dominant follicle and the initiation of a new follicular phase for recruitment and selection of a new dominant follicle (Collins and Hodgen 1986).

Ovulation occurs between 24 and 36 hours after the start of the LH surge, and the timing of oocyte retrieval for IVF can therefore be assessed in relation to changes in both LH and progesterone.

2.3   Stimulated Follicular Development

Gonadotrophin administration is a highly successful form of infertility treatment, offering pregnancy rates similar to those in the normal fertile population (Hull et al. 1979; Healy et al. 1980; West and Baird 1984; Diamond and Wentz 1986). The major drawbacks to such treatment are hyperstimulation (see below) and multiple pregnancy. However, in the context of IVF, the latter situation is controlled by the transfer of a limited number of embryos.

The aim of follicular stimulation in an IVF programme is to increase the number of mature oocytes available for retrieval. Multiple oocyte aspiration not only improves the pregnancy success rate by permitting the transfer of more than one embryo, but it also allows for the subsequent return of the frozen–thawed embryos, thereby further augmenting the pregnancy rate per stimulated cycle (Trounson and Mohr 1983).

Theoretically, multiple ovulation can be achieved by either increasing the synchronous development of 2–4 mm antral follicles, or by extending the follicular phase FSH "gate" (Baird 1987). Although the former mechanism may be utilized in some breeds of sheep (Scaramuzzi and Radford 1983), most other means of improving the ovulation rate rely upon widening the FSH "gate".

Following the initial report of multiple follicular development for IVF using CC and hCG (Trounson et al. 1981), a number of stimulation regimens have now been described. These include CC alone (Wood et al. 1981; Trounson and Leeton 1982; Fishel et al. 1984), hMG (Jones et al. 1982; Laufer et al. 1983), CC plus hMG (Trounson, 1983), purified FSH (Jones 1985); Bernardus et al. 1985) and pulsatile gonadotrophin releasing hormone (GnRH) (Liu et al. 1983; Jones et al. 1986). Monitoring of ovarian stimulation during these treatments is usually performed using a combination of plasma oestradiol measurement and ovarian ultrasound.

In the Monash University IVF programme, information from the patient's six previous natural cycles is computed to calculate the expected mid-point and 95% confidence limits for the next cycle (McIntosh et al. 1980). CC is then given at a dose of 100 mg daily for 5 days, commencing 10 days prior to the anticipated mid-point. hMG administration – 150 IU daily – is started the day after the clomiphene and continues until the plasma oestradiol reaches between 500 and 1000 pg/ml. The duration and the daily dosage of hMG treatment is adjusted depending on the patient's individual response as judged by serum oestradiol and ovarian ultrasound determinations. Endocrine results are reviewed at a clinical meeting each afternoon when the subsequent day's stimulation is decided.

Once the serum oestradiol reaches between 800 and 1000 pg/ml, patients are admitted to hospital for more intensive monitoring. Blood is taken three times daily for oestradiol, progesterone and LH estimation and gonadotrophin treatment continues until the oestradiol concentration reaches about 300–500 pg/ml per 18 mm follicle. It is unusual to administer hMG once the confidence limits have been entered, although it is sometimes given if the oestradiol level suddenly declines. If a surge in plasma LH has not occurred within 36 hours of the predicted mid-point, 5000 IU of hCG are given, and oocyte retrieval is performed 36 hours later.

Analysis of the oestradiol response to stimulation has provided a practical method of assessing the progress of the treatment cycle. Collating data from 102

IVF conception cycles following standard stimulation regimens, the 5th and 95th centiles for plasma oestradiol on each day of treatment have been calculated (Fig. 2.2), enabling the objective diagnosis of both ovarian hyperstimulation and inadequate stimulation (Okamoto et al. 1986).

Although peripheral oestradiol is widely used to assess follicular growth this provides an index of thecal rather than granulosa cell function (McNatty et al. 1979). However, the recent characterization of inhibin has offered the chance of monitoring granulosa cell activity more specifically (Mason et al. 1985; Forage et al. 1986). A direct correlation has been demonstrated in plasma between inhibin and oestradiol concentrations in women undergoing hyperstimulation for IVF (McLachlan et al. 1986b).

2.3.1 Hyperstimulation

Ovarian hyperstimulation comprises a syndrome ranging from an increase in oestradiol and progesterone secretion in the absence of clinical symptoms, through varying degrees of ovarian enlargement and associated discomfort, with the most severe cases experiencing increases in blood viscosity, electrolyte imbalances and hypovolaemic shock (Rabau et al. 1967). Excessive ovarian hyperstimulation can cause death (Mozes et al. 1965; Schenker and Weinstein 1978).

Hyperstimulation is less common in hypogonadotrophic women than in individuals with normal FSH and LH concentrations (Lunenfeld and Insler 1974). The majority of patients undergoing IVF stimulation regimens have regular ovulatory cycles, yet ovarian hyperstimulation remains relatively infrequent despite the development of multiple follicles and high oestradiol levels. The main difference between IVF stimulation and ovulation induction with gonadotrophins, however, is that in the former situation oocyte retrieval offers the opportunity to puncture all significant follicles thereby reducing the incidence of this potentially serious syndrome.

2.3.2 Inadequate Stimulation

About 20% of patients who commence IVF superovulation treatment are discharged before oocyte recovery (Jones 1985). Reasons for abandoning treatment vary between different IVF centres and include not only biological factors such as low plasma oestradiol concentrations, but also organizational difficulties such as the presence of a spontaneous LH rise in women attending clinics where out of hours egg collection is not possible.

There are three clinical choices when faced with unsatisfactory stimulation. Firstly, the couple can be discharged from further attempts at IVF. Secondly, the stimulation regimen can be repeated in a few months time in the hope of spontaneous improvement. Finally, a natural menstrual cycle can be assessed in order to devise a more appropriate stimulation in the next IVF attempt. Mere repetition of the same superovulation regimen results in improved folliculogenesis in only 10% of patients (D. L. Healy, unpublished data).

As it remains unclear why not all women with regular menstrual cycles respond to IVF ovarian stimulation we have investigated consecutive patients at least 3

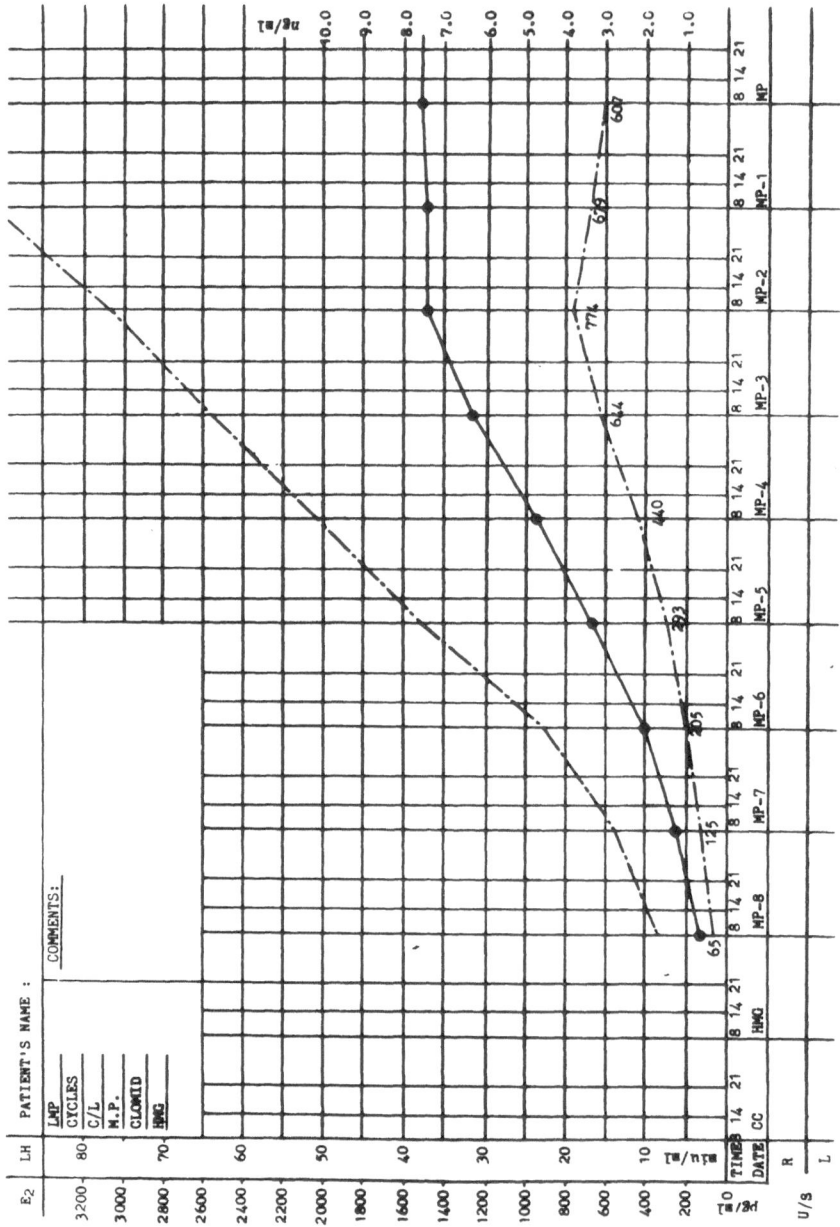

Fig. 2.2. Treatment cycle stimulation – oestradiol concentrations. The median, 5th and 95th centiles for 102 IVF conception cycles have been charted to define the limits of normal stimulation. MP, cycle mid-point.

months after a failed IVF attempt. Two-thirds of the treatment cycles had been cancelled because of inadequate oestradiol concentrations. A weekly blood sample was taken from day 1 on a spontaneous menstrual cycle and assayed for FSH, LH, prolactin, oestradiol and progesterone concentrations (O'Shea et al. 1986). Of 131 spontaneous menstrual cycles 47 (36%) were considered endocrinologically normal. The remaining 84 (64%) revealed the following abnormalities:

1. Low luteal phase progesterone (peak progesterone <6 ng/ml) $n = 33$.
2. Premature progesterone elevation (progesterone concentration >5 ng/ml on day 15) $n = 27$.
3. Occult ovarian failure (early follicular phase FSH >30 U/l) $n = 14$.
4. Early follicular phase LH:FSH ratio >3, $n = 6$.
5. Hyperprolactinaemia (prolactin >30 ng/ml) $n = 4$.

2.3.2.1 Premature Progesterone Elevation

Although serum progesterone concentrations were normal in the mid-luteal phase, levels were elevated as early as day 15 of the spontaneous cycle. This suggests that ovulation occurred on day 10 or 11 and that follicle selection may also have taken place at a correspondingly premature stage of the cycle. If this hypothesis is true, then the early commencement of ovarian stimulation may result in the recruitment of a larger group of synchronous antral follicles.

2.3.2.2 Occult Ovarian Failure

We have defined this condition as the occurrence of elevated plasma FSH concentrations in the presence of regular menstrual cycles (Fig. 2.3). It is possible

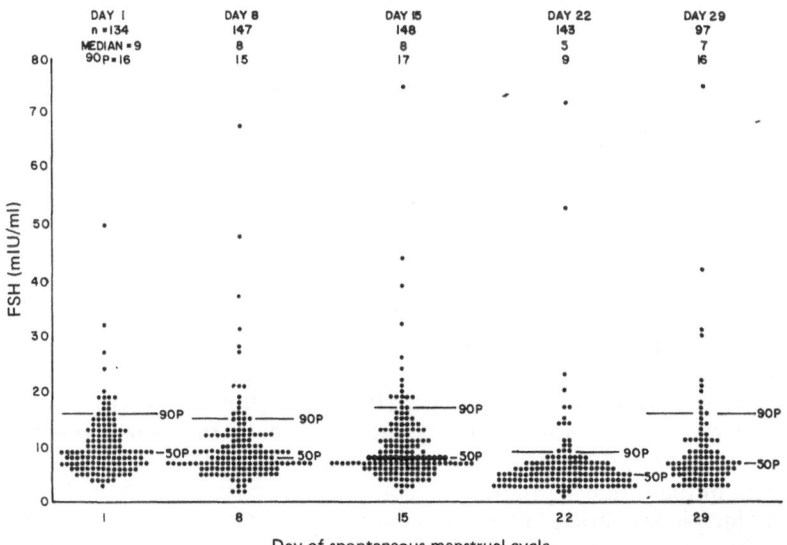

Fig. 2.3 Serum FSH concentrations (U/l) during spontaneous menstrual cycles from women under treatment in the Monash IVF programme.

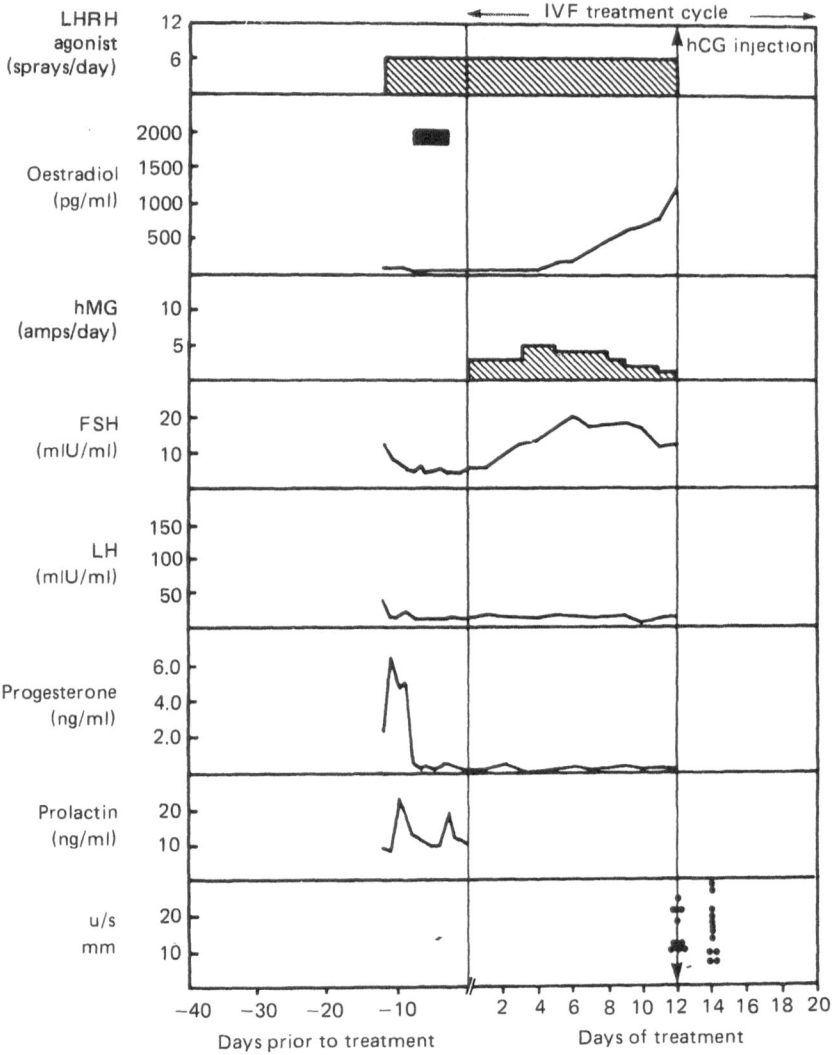

Fig. 2.4. Buserelin and hMG for the IVF treatment cycle. U/S, follicular diameters (mm) on vaginal ultrasound assessment.

that occult ovarian failure could represent an early stage of premature ovarian failure (Board et al. 1979); however, further studies are required to define the relationship between occult ovarian failure and the detection of autoantibodies and other stigmata of ovarian failure proper (Irvine and Barnes 1974).

The optimal method of ovarian hyperstimulation in these women remains undecided. Commencing IVF treatment at an earlier stage of the cycle has not been successful in the Monash programme. Likewise, in a similar group of eight women with "incipient ovarian failure" in whom ovarian stimulation had failed, the use of GnRH to stimulate follicular development resulted in successful oocyte aspiration in only two cases, though the transfer of a subsequent 6-cell embryo led to the birth of a normal girl (Jones et al. 1986).

2.3.3   GnRH Agonists

Elevated plasma LH concentrations may result in failed IVF stimulation because of thecal androgen-impaired folliculogenesis (Stanger and Yovich 1985). One approach to improve ovarian hyperstimulation in such cases could be to effect CC/hMG stimulation after pituitary down-regulation with one of the GnRH agonists (Fleming et al. 1986; McLachlan et al. 1986a).

The administration of intra-nasal buserelin (D-Ser3-^{t}Bu^6-EA^{10}-LHRH, Hoechst AG, Frankfurt) has been investigated in 44 women in whom previous attempts at IVF had failed to obtain more than one oocyte (MacLachlan et al. 1987). The median number of oocytes retrieved from 29 patients receiving buserelin and hMG was 4 (range 0,19), with 0 (0,5) being obtained from women treated with standard CC/hMG. The fertilization rate was 76% in each group. Of women receiving buserelin and hMG, 84% underwent the transfer of three embryos whereas this was only true of 13% of the CC/hMG group. A total of three pregnancies ensued, all from triple embryo transfers and all in the buserelin-treated women. An example of the endocrine profile resulting from hMG stimulation after buserelin for IVF is shown in Fig. 2.4. These data suggest that in appropriately selected patients, the use of a GnRH agonist to induce hypogonadotrophism is of benefit in a subsequent IVF attempt. Supplementary studies are required to assess whether the use of such agonists in standard IVF stimulation regimens will also lead to synchronous folliculogenesis with the retrieval of a larger number of oocytes.

2.4   Conclusion

In the Monash IVF programme no more than eight eggs are fertilized per treatment cycle and a maximum of three or four embryos are transferred some 48 hours later. The overall objective of stimulation, therefore, is to obtain between three and eight mature oocytes. A better understanding of the control of normal folliculogenesis and the increasing availability of alternative means for ovarian stimulation should lead to an improved ability to recruit a synchronous cohort of follicles to achieve this objective.

References

Baird DT (1983) Factors regulating the growth of the preovulatory follicle in the sheep and human. J Reprod Fertil 69:343–352

Baird DT (1987) A model for follicular selection and ovulation: lessons from superovulation. J Steroid Biochem 27:15–23

Baird DT, Fraser IS (1975) Concentration of oestrone and oestradiol 17β in follicular fluid and ovarian venous blood of women. Clin Endocrinol 4:259–266

Baird DT, Backstrom T, McNeilly AS, Smith SK, Wathen CG (1984) Effect of enucleation of the corpus luteum at different stages of the luteal phase of the human menstrual cycle on subsequent follicular development. J Reprod Fertil 70:615–624

Baker TG (1963) A quantitative and cytological study of germ cells in human ovaries. Proc R Soc Lond 158:417–433

Bernardus RE, Jones GS, Acosta AA, et al. (1985) The significance of the ratio in follicle-stimulating hormone and luteinizing hormone in induction of multiple follicular growth. Fertil Steril 43:373–379

Board JA, Redwine FO, Moncure CW, Frable WJ, Taylor JR (1979) Identification of differing etiologies of clinically diagnosed premature menopause. Am J Obstet Gynecol 134:939–943

Brown JB (1978) Pituitary control of ovarian function – concepts derived from gonadotrophin therapy. Aust NZ J Obstet Gynaecol 18:47–54

Collins RL, Hodgen GD (1986) Blockade of the spontaneous midcycle gonadotrophin surge in monkeys by RU486: a progesterone antagonist or agonist? J Clin Endocrinol Metab 63:1270–1276

Diamond MP, Wentz AC (1986) Ovulation induction with human menopausal gonadotropins. Obstet Gynecol Surv 41:480–490

diZerega GS, Hodgen GD (1980) Cessation of folliculogenesis during the primate luteal phase. J Clin Endocrinol Metab 51:158–160

Findlay JK (1986) The nature of inhibin and its use in the regulation of fertility and diagnosis of infertility. Fertil Steril 46:770–783

Fishel SB, Edwards RG, Purdy JM (1984) Analysis of infertile patients treated consecutively by in vitro fertilisation at Bourn Hall. Fertil Steril 42:191–193

Fleming R, Coutts JRT (1986) Induction of multiple follicular growth in normally menstruating women with endogenous gonadotrophin suppression. Fertil Steril 45:226–230

Forage RG., Ring JM, Brown RW et al. (1986) Cloning and sequence analysis of cDNA species coding for the two sub-units of inhibin from bovine follicular fluid. Proc Natl Acad Sci USA 83:3091–3095

Garcia JE, Jones GS, Acosta AA, Wright G (1983) Human menopausal gonadotrophin/human chorionic gonadotrophin follicular maturation for oocyte aspiration: Phase 1, 1981. Fertil Steril 39:167–171

Goodman AL, Hodgen GD (1983) The ovarian triad of the primate menstrual cycle. Recent Prog Horm Res 39:1–67

Goodman AL, Nixon WE, Johnson DK, Hodgen GD (1977) Regulation of folliculogenesis in the cycling Rhesus monkey: selection of the dominant follicle. Endocrinology 100:155–161

Healy DL, Kovacs GT, Pepperell RJ, Burger HG (1980) A normal cumulative conception rate after human pituitary gonadotrophin. Fertil Steril 34:341–345

Hodgen GD (1982) The dominant ovarian follicle. Fertil Steril 38:281–300

Hull MGR, Savage PE, Jacobs HS (1979) Investigation and treatment of amenorrhoea resulting in normal fertility. Br Med J i:1257–1261

Irvine WJ, Barnes EW (1974) Addison's disease and autoimmune ovarian failure. J Reprod Fertil [Suppl] 21:1–33

Jones GS (1985) Use of purified gonadotrophins for ovarian stimulation in IVF. In: Wood EC, Trounson AO (eds) New clinical issues in in vitro fertilisation. Saunders, London pp 775–784

Jones GS, Garcia JE, Rosenwaks Z (1984) The role of pituitary gonadotrophins in follicular stimulation and oocyte maturation in the human. J Clin Endocrinol Metab 59:178–180

Jones GS, Muasher SJ, Rosenwaks Z, Acosta AA, Liu HC (1986) The perimenopausal patient in in vitro fertilisation: the use of gonadotrophin-releasing hormone. Fertil Steril 46:885–891

Jones HW, Jones GS, Andrews MC et al. (1982) The program for in vitro fertilisation at Norfolk. Fertil Steril 38:14–21

Jones HW, Acosta AA, Andrews MC et al. (1983) The importance of follicular phase to success and failure of in vitro fertilisation. Fertil Steril 40:317–321

Laufer N, deCherney AH, Haseltine FP et al. (1983) The use of high-dose human menopausal gonadotrophin in an in vitro fertilisation program. Fertil Steril 40:734–737

Leyendecker G, Wildt L, Gips H, Nocke W, Pletz EJ (1976) Experimental studies on the positive feedback of progesterone, 17α-hydroxyprogesterone and 20α-dihydroprogesterone on the pituitary release of LH and FSH in the human female. Arch Gynecol 221:29–45

Liu JH, Durfee RD, Muse K, Yen SSC (1983) Induction of multiple ovulation by pulsatile administration of gonadotrophin-releasing hormone. Fertil Steril 40:18–23

Lunenfeld B, Insler V (1974) Classification of amenorrhoeic states and their treatment by ovulation induction. Clin Endocrinol 3:223–237

McLachlan RI, Healy DL, Burger HG (1986a) Clinical aspects of LHRH analogues in gynaecology: a review. Br J Obstet Gynaecol 93:431–454

McLachlan RI, Robertson DM, Healy DL, deKretser DM, Burger HG (1986b) Plasma inhibin levels during gonadotrophin-induced ovarian hyperstimulation for IVF: a new index of follicular function? Lancet I:1233–1234

MacLachlan VB, Besanko MD, Wade HD et al. (1987) Controlled trial of clomiphene citrate (CC)–human menopausal gonadotropin (hMG) or buserelin–hMG treatment in previously resistant IVF patients. Proc Endocr Soc Aust 30:29

Mason AJ, Hayflick JS, Ring N et al. (1985) Complementary DNA sequences of ovarian follicular fluid inhibin show precursor structure and homology with transforming growth factor-β. Nature 318:659–663

McIntosh JEA, Matthews CD, Crocker JM, Broom TJ, Cox LW (1980) Predicting the luteinizing hormone surge: relationship between the duration of the follicular and the luteal phases and the length of the human menstrual cycle. Fertil Steril 34:125–130

McNatty KP, Makris A, de Grazia C, Osathamondh R, Ryan KJ (1979) The production of progesterone androgen and oestrogens by granulosa cells, thecal tissue and stromal tissue from human ovaries in vitro. J Clin Endocrinol Metab 49:687–699

McNatty KP, Hillier SG, van den Boogard AMJ, Trimbos-Kemper TCM, Reichert LE Jnr, van Hall EV (1983) Follicular development during the luteal phase of the human menstrual cycle. J Clin Endocrinol Metab 56:1022–1031

Mozes M, Bogokowsky H, Antebi E et al. (1965) Thromboembolic phenomena after ovarian stimulation with human menopausal gonadotrophins. Lancet II:1213–1215

Nillius SJ, Wide L (1971) Induction of a midcycle-like peak of luteinizing hormone in young women by exogenous oestradiol-17β. Br J Obstet Gynaecol 78:822–827

Nilsson L, Wikland M, Hamburger L (1982) Recruitment of an ovulatory follicle in the human following follicle-ectomy and lute-ectomy. Fertil Steril 37:30–34

Odell WD, Swerdloff RS (1968) Progesterone-induced luteinizing and follicle stimulating hormone surge in postmenopausal women: a simulated ovulatory peak. Proc Natl Acad Sci USA 51:529–536

Okamoto S, Healy DL, Howlett DT et al. (1986) An analysis of plasma oestradiol concentrations during clomiphene citrate–human menopausal gonadotrophin stimulation in an in vitro fertilisation–embryo transfer program. J Clin Endocrinol Metab 63:736–740

Ono T, Campeau JD, Holmberg EA et al. (1986) Biochemical and physiologic characterisation of follicle regulatory protein: a paracrine regulator of folliculogenesis. Am J Obstet Gynecol 154:709–716

O'Shea FC, Healy DL, Besanko MD et al. (1986) Unsatisfactory superovulation responses in IVF: classification and endocrine assessment of a subsequent spontaneous menstrual cycle. Proc Fert Soc Aust: A4 abstract

Rabau E, David A, Serr DM, Maschiach S, Lunenfeld B (1967) Human menopausal gonadotrophins for anovulation and sterility. Results of 7 years of treatment. Am J Obstet Gynecol 98:92–98

Rogers P, Molloy D, Healy D et al. (1986) Cross-over trial of superovulation protocols from two major in vitro fertilisation centres. Fertil Steril 46:424–431

Ross GT, van de Wiele RL (1981) The ovary. In: Williams R (ed) Textbook of endocrinology, 6th edn. Saunders, Philadelphia pp 355–399

Scaramuzzi RJ, Radford HM (1983) Factors regulating ovulation rate in the ewe. J Reprod Fertil 69:353–357

Schenken RS, Werlin LB, Williams RF, Prihoda TJ, Hodgen GD (1985) Periovulatory hormonal dynamics: relationship of immunoassayable gonadotrophins and ovarian steroids to the bioassayable luteinizing hormone surge in rhesus monkeys. J Clin Endocrinol Metab 60:886–890

Schenker JG, Weinstein D (1978) Ovarian hyperstimulation syndrome: a current survey. Fertil Steril 30:255–268

Stanger JD, Yovich JL (1985) Reduced in vitro fertilisation of human oocytes from patients with raised basal luteinizing hormone levels during the follicular phase. Br J Obstet Gynaecol 92:385–393

Trounson AO (1983) In vitro fertilisation at Monash University, Melbourne, Australia. In: Crosignani PG, Rubin, BL (eds) In vitro fertilisation and embryo transfer. Academic Press, New York pp 315–322

Trounson AO, Leeton JF (1982) The endocrinology of clomiphene stimulation. In: Edwards RG, Purdy JM (eds) Human conception in vitro. Academic Press, New York pp 51–70

Trounson AO, Mohr L (1983) Human pregnancy following cryopreservation, thawing and transfer of an 8-cell embryo. Nature 305:707–709

Trounson AO, Leeton JF, Wood EC, Webb J, Wood J (1981) Pregnancies in humans by fertilisation in vitro and embryo transfer in the controlled ovulatory cycle. Science 212:681–682

West CP, Baird DT (1984) Induction of ovulation with gonadotrophins – a ten year review. Scott Med
    J 29:212–217
Wood C, Trounson AO, Leeton JF et al. (1981) A clinical assessment of nine pregnancies obtained by
    in vitro fertilisation and embryo transfer. Fertil Steril 35:502–507

3 Oocyte Pick-up

J. Leeton

3.1 Introduction

Both the indications for and success rates of in vitro fertilization (IVF) programmes have steadily increased during the last few years in most centres, but the actual number of programmes throughout the world has greatly increased. Although many clinics now claim an overall pregnancy rate of 15%–30% per egg retrieval procedure, the cost of the programmes remains relatively high. Technical improvements in limiting costs are mandatory to meet the rising demand for this technique. The major cost in many IVF programmes is related to the time spent in hospital, which is dependent upon the type of anaesthesia, recovery time, degree of invasiveness of the procedure and risks involved. No fundamental changes have been introduced into general IVF programmes during the last few years in the areas of ovarian stimulation, IVF techniques and embryo transfer (ET) procedures. However, the new methods of egg collection using ultrasonic techniques are now being rapidly developed in many centres. Their main advantages compared with the older laparoscopic technique lie in their associated reduction in cost of the egg collection procedure due to reduced hospitalization stay and better acceptance by the patient without reducing the effectiveness of the egg collection rate.

3.2 Laparoscopic Method

The laparoscopic method remains the most common method of egg collection in many clinics today but is rapidly being replaced by the newer ultrasonic methods. No further significant data regarding the laparoscopic method are available since its description in the first edition of this book. It remains an effective and safe technique of obtaining oocytes from stimulated and accessible ovaries with a 70%–90% egg collection rate per follicle. Debate continues regarding the optimum needle diameter, preference for single or two-way needle systems, the importance of the skill and technique of the operator, the need to flush follicles and the type of anaesthesia used. Although the incidence of serious or adverse side effects with this method is extremely low, its main disadvantage lies in the necessary use of general anaesthesia, the limitation of access to adherent or covered ovaries and its common post-operative abdominal discomfort and hospitalization stay of 6–24 hours. In all these regards the ultrasound procedures have a definite advantage.

3.3   Ultrasound-Guided Techniques

3.3.1   Transvesical Approach

The collection of human oocytes for IVF by ultrasound-guided percutaneous follicular puncture was first described by Lenz in 1981 (Lenz et al. 1981). This was a natural development based on the previous knowledge of ultrasound-guided punctures of other abdominal organs. In the following year further reports on the successful use of ultrasonically-guided percutaneous oocyte aspiration were made (Lenz and Lauritsen 1982; Wickland et al. 1983; Hamberger et al. 1982). These workers, using abdominal transducers with frequencies between 3.5 and 5.0 MHz, encountered difficulty sometimes in visualizing poorly stimulated ovaries especially in obese patients. Filling the urinary bladder with a volume of 300–500 ml generally gave better visualization and was routinely used. This transvesical aspiration route utilizing an abdominal transducer equipped with an attached needle guide is still used in some IVF centres today. Its main disadvantages lie in the difficulty of performing this procedure with local anaesthesia since the bladder wall remains sensitive in many cases to needle puncture, and filling of the bladder with up to 500 ml, which usually causes a significant degree of patient discomfort. This method requires a degree of training and experience in ultrasound techniques by the operator before satisfactory oocyte collection rates can be achieved.

3.3.2   Perurethral Approach

The perurethral approach requires the passage of a needle through the urethra into a filled bladder under control of an abdominal transducer (Parsons et al. 1985). Good egg recovery rates have been obtained but again a degree of training over several months in ultrasound is usually required.

3.3.3   Transvaginal Approach

The transvaginal route of follicular aspiration using an abdominal transducer to visualize the ovaries was first described by Dellenbach and co-workers in 1984 and by Wickland and colleagues in 1985. This technique also required a full urinary bladder which was therefore associated with discomfort to the patient and often difficulty in visualizing ovarian follicles particularly those of smaller diameter. Wickland's original report quoted an oocyte collection rate of 36%. The free-hand puncture technique described in his earlier reports usually required a significant degree of ultrasonic skill and experience of lining up the abdominal transducer with the vaginal needle.

A more direct and easier method entailed passing the needle along the line of an ultrasonic transducer which was designed for introduction into the vagina. This new modification was first reported in 1984 (Wickland et al. 1985) and since then several publications describing both the simplicity and effectiveness of this technique have been reported (Feichtinger and Kameter 1986; Cohen et al. 1986; Torode et al. 1986; Lenz et al. 1987). This method is now the optimal technique for obtaining oocytes for IVF as it possesses distinct advantages over previously described methods of ultrasonically-guided egg collection. These include a minimum risk of morbidity especially trauma to the bladder, greater accuracy of location of follicles due to their closer proximity to the transducer element, the opportunity of carrying out the procedure under local anaesthesia or light intravenous sedation, and the ease with which the method can be learnt quickly by clinicians without previous experience with ultrasonic techniques (Lenz et al. 1987).

3.4   Ultrasound-Guided Technique Using a Combined Vaginal Needle and Transducer

3.4.1   Machines

Several ultrasound machines equipped with vaginal transducers are now available and their number is increasing. The ultrasound scanner used in our IVF programme is a General Electric RT3000 with a vaginal 5 MHz curved array puncture transducer. For puncture procedures it is necessary to have an accurately aligned needle guide which requires minimum space in the vagina, so that the combined transducer and needle guide can be introduced into the vagina without discomfort (Fig. 3.1).

3.4.2   Aspiration Needles

Aspiration needles used in our programme are made of stainless steel with a length of 31 cm and an internal diameter of 1.15 mm. The tips must be extremely sharp to enable puncture of mobile ovaries and must therefore be disposable. They are usually introduced through the vaginal vault with a sharp internal stylet which is withdrawn immediately the ovarian capsule is punctured. The needle is connected to tubing which collects the follicular fluid under pressure of 120–150 mmHg from a suction pump; the method is similar to those described previously for laparoscopic oocyte collection (Renou et al. 1981).

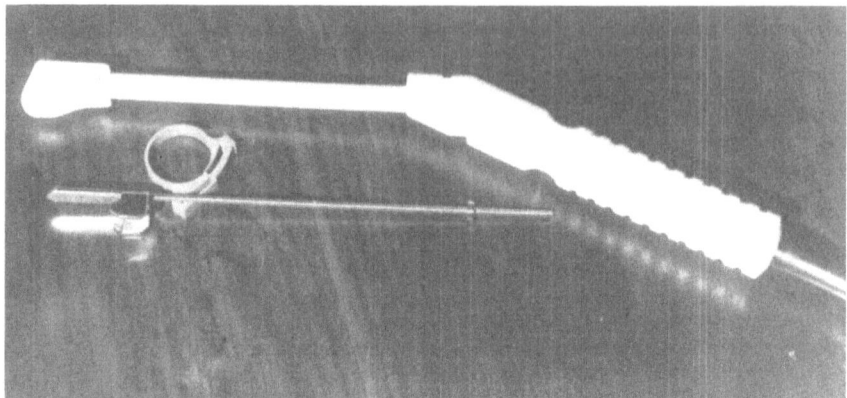

Fig. 3.1. A 5.0 MHz vaginal sector transducer with fixed puncture attachment.

3.4.3   Sterilization of Transducers

As it is deleterious to sterilize the transducer because of the risk of damage to the transducer element or casing, it has been found adequate to enclose the transducer probe in either a sterile bag, condom or surgical glove prior to insertion into the vagina. The transducer is carefully washed in water following each procedure.

3.4.4   Vaginal Preparation

The vagina need only be swabbed with sterile saline, particularly in the fornices; disinfectants should not be used because of possible toxic effects on the oocytes. Antibiotic cover is not necessary and no clinical infections have been noted in our series of over 800 procedures using this protocol.

3.4.5   Anaesthesia

Premedication and general anaesthesia may be used as for routine laparoscopy. Paracervical block with 10 ml 1% lidocaine and mild intravenous sedation can give good local anaesthesia with patients remaining coherent throughout the procedure (Russell et al. 1987). Our IVF programme has successfully used varying combinations of neurolept anaesthesia where several short-acting narcotics are administered by intravenous infusion. Patient compliance, good analgesia and rapid recovery have been found in most procedures, but patients' preferences should be considered in the final choice of anaesthesia.

3.4.6   Technique

Prior to puncture of the vault and ovaries with the needle, both ovaries should be carefully scanned to check the size and position of their follicles. The guideline on the television screen is placed by adjustment of the transducer so that it crosses the maximum diameter of the follicle to be punctured thus ensuring needle puncture at right angles to the follicular wall (Fig. 3.2). It is generally useful to (1) aspirate follicles from a lateral to medial direction so that an orderly sequence is maintained, (2) aspirate the larger follicles (>18 mm diameter) first as these are most likely to contain the more mature oocytes, and (3) aspirate deeper follicles before superficial ones as leakage and bleeding from the latter can disfigure the ultrasound image by either shadowing or reflection artifacts.

The needle and stylet are usually introduced into the first follicle after which the stylet is withdrawn and the suction tubing immediately applied to the end of the needle to ensure that leakage of fluid does not occur. The follicle is seen to

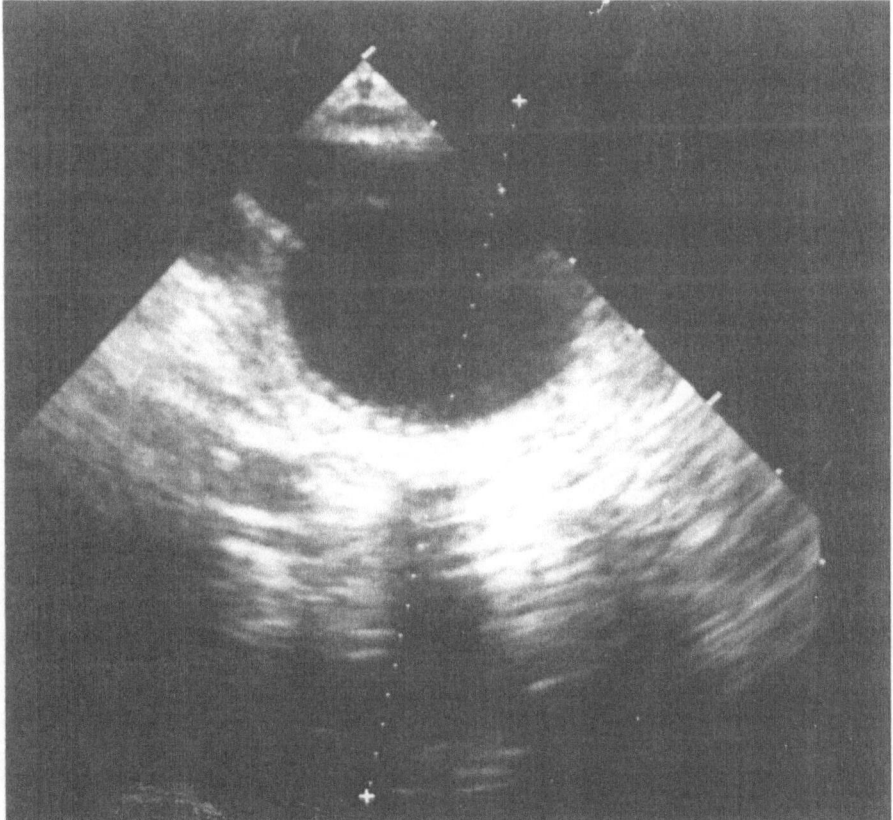

Fig. 3.2.   Scan image of two stimulated ovarian follicles with superimposed puncture guideline.

rapidly empty on the screen, which should be constantly observed by the operator (Fig. 3.3). During follicle aspiration the needle should be rotated and moved gently in all directions around the inner circumference of the follicle to give a curettage effect which increases the chance of oocyte collection. If the oocyte is not recovered in the first aspirate, flushing the follicle may be carried out several times by disconnecting the bung and injecting culture medium into the tubing using a needle and syringe as described for laparoscopic egg collection (Wood et al. 1981). Some operators do not flush follicles and claim a high oocyte collection rate from a single aspiration. Flushing of follicles is unlikely to produce a mature oocyte beyond the fourth flush but several flushings can be carried out quickly over a period of only 1 or 2 minutes.

Once an oocyte is obtained from the follicle the needle can be carefully withdrawn and lined up opposite a neighbouring follicle without necessarily removing the needle from the ovarian surface. Puncturing of the external follicular surface will often produce discomfort in the unanaesthetised patient. In

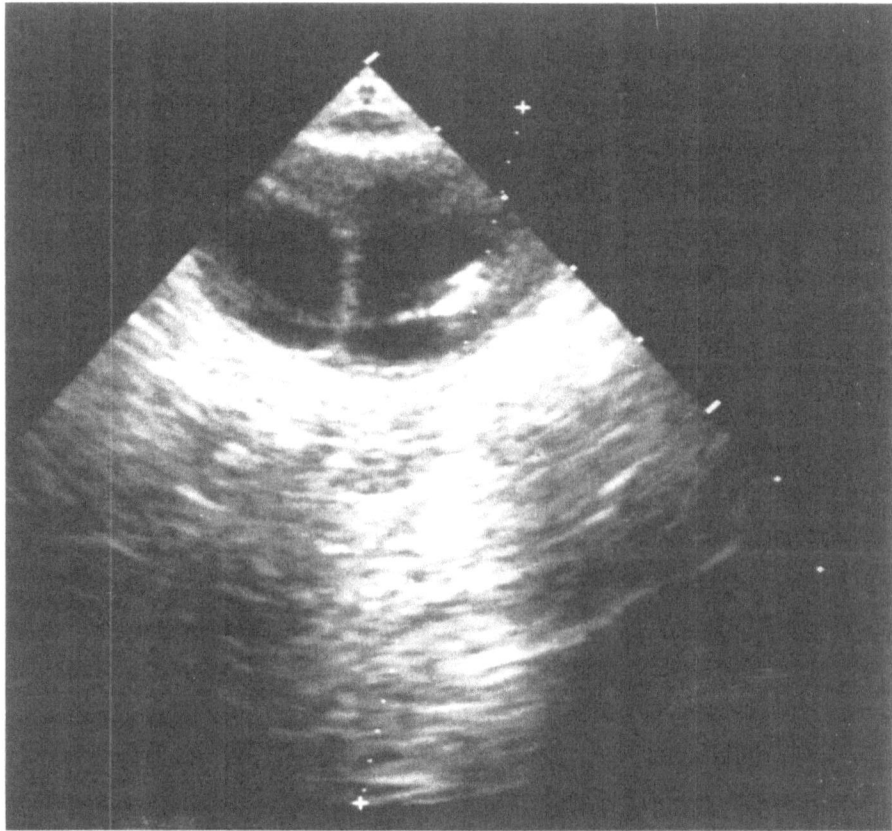

Fig. 3.3. Scan image of the same follicles with visible needle-tip echo in the centre of the larger follicle which is undergoing aspiration and collapse.

this method several follicles may be rapidly aspirated from one ovary without withdrawing the needle. When aspirating the opposite ovary the needle must be withdrawn as the transducer probe usually requires positioning in a new direction in the opposite vaginal fornix. The needle with its stylet is then introduced through the vaginal vault to aspirate the opposite ovary as described above. Following the oocyte collection the vagina is gently swabbed with sterile saline. The whole procedure usually takes no longer than 30 minutes and the patient is fit to leave the clinic within 4 hours if general anaesthesia has not been used.

3.4.7 Difficulties with Technique

Surprisingly few difficulties have been encountered with this transvaginal technique. Difficulty in puncturing mobile ovaries can usually be overcome by the use of sharp needles and the employment of a sharp stabbing motion by the operator. Small bowel is rarely seen between the vaginal vault and the ovary and can usually be avoided by redirection of the transducer. Occasionally the uterus lies between the vaginal vault and the ovary making ovarian aspiration difficult. This can usually be overcome by positioning the ovary by manual pressure on the abdomen, rotation and redirection of the transducer, or occasionally reaching the ovary by passing the needle directly through the uterus. The latter procedure appears to have minimal risk of damage or bleeding. It is surprising what little bleeding and trauma is seen following vaginal needling of the ovaries when checked by laparoscopic examination immediately following the procedure. Pelvic adhesions and fixed pelvic structures offer no restriction to the vaginal method and in fact enhance the chance of egg collection by nature of the ovarian fixity. There has been no case of morbidity, including significant internal or external bleeding, in our experience of over 800 procedures. Several cases of moderate bleeding from the vaginal vault have been controlled by packing the vaginal fornix. Where suspected ovulation has occurred fluid from the pouch of Douglas can be easily visualized and aspirated with this vaginal approach.

3.5 Results

Most groups using laparoscopic techniques reported oocyte recovery rates of approximately 90% (Renou et al. 1981). Originally oocyte collection rates employing the transvaginal method were significantly reduced (Wickland et al. 1985). Recent reports, however, have confirmed an egg collection rate and pregnancy rate comparable to those found in IVF programmes employing laparoscopic egg collection techniques (Torode et al. 1986; Feichtinger and Kameter 1986; Hamberger et al. 1986; Lewin et al. 1986). Our own results are described in Table 3.1. These results show comparable findings between laparoscopic and ultrasonically controlled techniques of egg collection although the two groups were not matched. The relatively low egg collection rate per follicle with the ultrasonic method was largely related to the learning curve of the clinicians, none of whom had previous experience with ultrasonic techniques (Lenz et al. 1987).

Table 3.1.   Vaginal ultrasound vs. laparoscopic technique for oocyte collection (Kovacs et al. 1987)

	Vaginal ultrasound	Laparoscopy
Procedures	609	139
No. follicles aspirated	5168	991
Median (range)	9 (1–44)	8 (1–20)
No. eggs retrieved	3170	710
Median (range)	6 (0–25)	6 (0–15)
% eggs recovered per follicles aspirated	61%[a]	72%[a]
Fertilization rate	64% (1864/2902)	66% (402/607)
Pregnancies per egg pick-up	78[b] (13%)	23[b] (17%)

[a] $\chi^2 = 2.2$; $P>0.05$, NS.
[b] $\chi^2 = 2.4$; $P>0.05$, NS.

3.6   Conclusions

The aspiration of oocytes from stimulated follicles using an ultrasound-guided technique with a vaginal needle and transducer has egg collection rates and pregnancy rates comparable to those of laparoscopic techniques. As the former technique also offers precise imaging of all ovarian follicles, minimum risk, limited discomfort, good patient compliance and quick recovery rate, it should be considered the optimum method of oocyte collection in all IVF programmes.

References

Cohen J, Debacte C, Pez JP, Junca AM, Cohen-Bacrie P (1986) Transvaginal sonographically controlled ovarian puncture for oocyte retrieval for IVF. J In Vitro Fert Embryo Transfer 3:309–313

Dellenbach P, Nisband I, Moreau L et al. (1984) Transvaginal sonographically controlled ovarian follicle puncture for egg retrieval. Lancet I:1467

Feichtinger W, Kameter P (1986) Laparoscopic or ultrasonically guided follicle aspiration for in vitro fertilization. J In Vitro Fert Embryo Transfer 1:244–249

Hamberger L, Wickland M, Nilsson L, Janson PO, Sjogren A, Hillensjo T (1982) Methods of aspiration of human oocytes by various techniques. Acta Med Rom 20:370–378

Hamberger L, Wickland M, Enk L, Nilsson L (1986) Laparoscopy versus ultrasound guided puncture for oocyte retrieval. Acta Eur Fertil 17:195–198

Kovacs G, King C, Cameron I et al. (1987) A comparison of vaginal ultrasonic-guided and laparoscopic retrieval of oocytes for in vitro fertilisation. In: Proceedings of the Fertility Society of Australia, 6th Scientific Meeting, Sydney, p 38

Lenz S, Lauritsen J (1982) Ultrasonically guided percutaneous aspiration of human follicles under local anaesthesia: a new method of collecting oocytes for in vitro fertilization. Fertil Steril 38:673–677

Lenz S, Lauritsen JG, Kjellow M (1981) Collection of human oocytes for in vitro fertilization by ultrasonically guided follicular puncture. Lancet I:1163

Lenz S, Leeton J, Renou P (1987) Transvaginal recovery of oocytes for IVF using vaginal ultrasound. J In Vitro Fert Embryo Transfer 4:51–55

Lewin A, Laufer N, Rabinowitz R, Margolioth EJ, Bar J, Schenker JG (1986) Ultrasonically-guided oocyte collection under local anaesthesia: the first choice method for in vitro fertilization – a comparative study with laparoscopy. Fertil Steril 46:257–261

Parsons J, Booker M, Goswamy R et al. (1985) Oocyte retrieval for in vitro fertilization by ultrasonically guided needle aspiration via the urethra. Lancet I:1076

Renou P, Trounson AO, Wood C, Leeton JF (1981) The collection of human oocytes for in vitro fertilization. An instrument for maximizing oocyte recovery rate. Fertil Steril 35:409–412

Russell JB, De Cherney AH, Hobbins JC (1987) A new transvaginal probe and biopsy guide for oocyte retrieval. Fertil Steril 47:350–352

Torode H, Picker R, Robertson R, Porter R, O'Neill C, Saunders D (1986) Initial results with transvaginal ultrasonically-guided oocyte pick-up in an Australian in vitro fertilization programme. Med J Aust 144:613–614

Wickland M, Nilsson L, Hansson R, Hamberger L, Jansen P (1983) Collection of human oocytes by the use of sonography. Fertil Steril 39:603–608

Wickland M, Enk L, Hamberger L (1985) Transvesical and transvaginal approaches for the aspiration of follicles by use of ultrasound. Ann NY Acad Sci 442:184–194

Wood C, Leeton JF, Talbot J Mc, Trounson AO (1981) Technique for collecting mature human oocytes for in vitro fertilization. Br J Obstet Gynaecol 88:756–760

4 Fertilization and Embryo Culture

A. Trounson

4.1 Introduction

Unlike many other mammalian species, human sperm capacitate in vitro and are capable of fertilizing eggs without being exposed to the female reproductive tract or requiring any special treatment to induce capacitation (Yanagimachi 1984). Separation of the motile sperm from the seminal plasma component of the ejaculate is easily achieved in most semen samples by centrifugation, washing and allowing sperm to swim from the spun pellet into overlayed culture medium (Mahadevan and Baker 1984). The addition of washed sperm to cultures containing mature human eggs results in dissolution of the cumulus oophorus through digestion of the hyaluronic acid matrix by sperm hyaluronidase, binding of sperm to the zona pellucida of the egg, penetration of the zona by acrosome reacted sperm and incorporation of the sperm into the egg cytoplasm within a few hours (McMaster et al. 1978; Sathananthan et al. 1985).

Although the preparation of sperm, insemination and culture of the eggs and early cleavage stage embryo is relatively simple, it is considered that this part of the in vitro fertilization (IVF) procedure is the one most likely to cause difficulty and correspondingly a reduction in the success rate of IVF. It is certainly the part most likely to be considered at fault when an IVF programme suffers a low success rate. However, it is often difficult to identify the specific problem because of our inability to measure embryo viability apart, that is, from the establishment of pregnancy following embryo replacement in vivo. In this chapter the general procedures for insemination of eggs and culture of embryos are described and an emphasis given to those aspects which may cause problems or which require careful control in order to prevent method drift into suboptimal conditions.

4.2 Quality Control of Laboratory Procedures

Basic quality control in the IVF laboratory is essential in order to maintain high fertilization rate and embryo viability. However, there is no simple quality control test that will guarantee that laboratory procedures are optimal. Essential laboratory control procedures which are simple but are frequently overlooked are discussed below.

4.2.1 Incubators

Incubators should be regularly cleaned and sterilized and this should be done following the manufacturers recommendation. Frequently alcohol vapour is used for sterilization. It is also advisable to examine regularly temperature variation in incubators using an independent thermocouple with a print out over 24 hours. It is not unusual for temperatures in some incubators to rise overnight to levels which are detrimental to cell viability. Few incubators are capable of cooling and in small rooms with no air conditioning or containing other heat emitting instruments, temperatures may exceed 37.5 °C. It is important to regularly check the control of CO_2 levels by adjustment of the CO_2 recording device using an independent instrument sampling from within the incubator. The maintenance of humidity in excess of 80% is also usually required for proper regulation of CO_2 controllers. When incubators are in frequent use it is advisable to ensure that the effects of variations in temperature, CO_2 levels and humidity are minimised by placing dishes or tubes containing eggs or embryos within desiccators or some other appropriate vessels within the incubator.

4.2.2 Glassware and Other Equipment

All glassware and other items which come into contact with culture medium, sperm, eggs or embryos should be washed and sterilized using tissue culture quality methods. All new glassware and tubing used for aspiration of eggs needs to be soaked in dilute acid solutions overnight, washed, ultrasonicated and adequately rinsed in pure water before use. When using detergents recommended for tissue culture ware, it is essential that the articles are rinsed properly in order to remove the detergents before sterilization. Dry heat sterilization is the most commonly used method for glassware, Teflon tubing and metal instruments used in IVF. If gas sterilization is used it is essential that the items are left long enough to allow all traces of gas to be removed. Autoclaving should not be used for sterilization and radiation is not recommended for all types of plastic because of toxic changes induced in the surfaces of some plastics.

4.2.3 Water

Water purity is very important for washing and rinsing tissue culture glassware and tubing and essential for the preparation for media used in IVF. Triple glass distilled water was the standard used for media preparation (Whittingham 1971) but more recently ultra-pure water produced by reverse osmosis and specialized filtration systems have replaced repeated distillation. While it has been reported (Fukuda et al. 1987) that fertilization rate, the proportion of fertilized eggs developing to blastocysts and the proportion of blastocysts hatching from the zona pellucida are directly related to the inorganic purity of water used to prepare culture medium (BWW medium, Biggers et al. 1971), others have shown that mouse embryos can develop quite readily in medium (Ham's F10) constituted from tap water (Silverman et al. 1987). However, neither of these studies examined embryo viability or their capacity to develop to fetuses when transferred to foster mothers. The conflicting results of the two studies illustrate the inadequacy of the culture of mouse embryos as a quality control system by itself.

Considerable care and attention is required to maintain ultra-pure water filtration systems. It is not sufficient to rely on measurement of electrical conductivity alone. These systems must be regularly sterilized and the water tested for organic contaminants, microorganisms and the presence of any other substances which can influence cell culture. If water purity can be relied on, it ceases to be a factor influencing the success of IVF, thus becoming an important quality control measure.

4.2.4 Other Factors

There are many other possible negative influences on cells grown in culture which require attention in the laboratory. It is not uncommon to identify one or more when trouble-shooting for IVF clinics with low pregnancy rates. While it is not possible to list every factor which should be examined, some examples may help in establishing the type of quality control required in each individual laboratory. Contamination of supposedly sterile plastic culture ware with microorganisms, including yeast and fungi, has occurred in some laboratories and a screening process of new batches of plastic culture ware is recommended. Serious contamination of incubators and whole laboratories has occurred from presumed sterile sources, risking the loss of all the eggs and embryos in culture at that time. On the other hand, some laboratories are zealously cleaned with volatile materials which by dissolving in culture solutions risk the loss of eggs and embryos. Heating blocks, warm stages and warm plates used to keep cells from cold shock, may overheat or may have hot spots on their surfaces. Temperatures in excess of 40 °C will irreversibly damage cells in mitosis and overheating of embryos must be avoided. It is important to check such warming instruments with surface thermocouples. Inadequately rinsed glass pipettes, used to handle embryos, may have detergent baked onto their surface after sterilization; this may then be transferred to cultures causing damage to embryos. The presence of baked-on detergent or other contaminating material should be suspected when pipettes packaged and sterilized together, stick to one another. This situation must be avoided. A simple test is to place washed pipettes in pure water for a short period of time, then vigorously shake the water. The formation of bubbles will demonstrate the presence of detergent.

4.2.5 Toxicity

The identification of toxic substances, used for culture or leaching from catheters and other instruments used in IVF, by the culture of mouse embryos in medium containing the material or rinses of the instruments, has been recommended for a long time (see Wood and Trounson 1982). This quality control model has been used to identify serious toxicity in culture components, catheters and other items

(Wood and Trounson 1982; Ackerman et al. 1984, 1985; Parinaud et al. 1987). While this test is helpful in determining whether new materials are seriously toxic to embryo development and should be used as a screen before introducing new materials into IVF, it is not the panacea for identifying suboptimal conditions which can affect embryo viability in human IVF. Toxicity of materials used in IVF can also be very simply determined using monolayer cell cultures and this is nicely demonstrated in the paper by Ray et al. (1987) who used amniotic fluid cells to identify the toxicity of different types of urethral catheters used in human IVF. This type of test could also be extremely useful for screening the introduction of new types of materials in IVF.

Routine quality control testing for more subtle effects which reduce embryo viability in vitro is more difficult. The screening of batches of culture medium by ascertaining the proportion of mouse embryos which develop from 2 cells to blastocyst is a rather insensitive test. We have explored a test involving cell cleavage kinetics of 2-cell mouse embryos. For this we measure the proportion of embryos at the 4-cell stage or 8-cell state in a given time. In suboptimal culture medium, cleavage rate will be slowed and fewer embryos will be at the expected cell stage at different intervals compared with embryos grown in optimal culture medium. This is a relatively simple and rapid test of culture media quality but data on its usefulness in human IVF has not been published to date. Culture media can also be screened by culture of other cell types (including selected hybridoma cells grown under serum free conditions) determining the time taken to confluency, cell number in culture wells after 2 to 4 days, mitotic index or some other measure of cell proliferation. However, no data exists on the merits for human IVF of selecting media using such tests.

4.3 Media for Insemination of Eggs and Culture of Embryos

A wide range of culture media have been used in human IVF. There is no consensus as to which is the best medium to use and there are very few properly controlled trials designed to assess culture media. The media used at present can be divided into those which are complex and contain many substances and those which consist of a simple balanced salt solution.

4.3.1 Complex Media

Complex tissue culture media made commercially is used for human IVF and is available as single strength liquid or 10 times concentrate. Some of the most widely used media in Europe are Menezo's B2 or B3 culture solutions (Table 1). B3 contains human serum albumin and does not require the addition of human serum for use (Menezo et al. 1984). Ham's F10 is also frequently used for IVF, particularly in North America, but this requires the addition of antibiotics and human serum (10 to 15%). It is of some concern that Ham's F10 contains hypoxanthine (Table 1) which has been shown to inhibit the development of embryos of some strains of mice in vitro (Loutradis et al. 1987). Under these

Table 4.1. Composition of complex media in use for human IVF

Ingredient	B2[a] (mg/l)	B3[b] (mg/l)	HF10[c] (mg/l)
NaCl	5 250	6 100	7 400
KCl	800	700	285
NaHCO$_3$	2 500	1 800	1 200
MgSO$_4$.7H$_2$O	200	200	152.8
Na$_2$HPO$_4$.12H$_2$O	154	154	290 (.7H$_2$O)
KH$_2$PO$_4$	60	60	83
Na acetate	50	50	—
Ca lactate	500	50	—
Na pyruvate	250	250	110
Serum albumin	10 000 (bovine)	10 000 (human)	—
Glucose	1 200	1 200	1 100
Phenol red	20	15	1.2
Vitamin C	50	50	—
Tween 80	50	—	—
Cholesterol	125	25	—
Penicillin	25 000 U	25 000 U	—
Streptomycin	40	40	—
CaCl$_2$.2H$_2$O	—	—	44.1
CuSO$_4$.5H$_2$O	—	—	0.0025
FeSO$_4$.7H$_2$O	—	—	0.834
ZnSO$_4$.7H$_2$O	—	—	0.0288
Lipoic acid	—	—	0.2
Thymidine	—	—	0.7
Hypoxanthine	—	—	4.0
pH	7.6	7.4	7.4
H$_2$O (mosmol/kg)	290	280	300

[a] Includes in addition amino acids (Menezo 1976).
[b] Includes in addition amino acids and other substances (Menezo et al. 1984).
[c] Includes in addition amino acids and vitamins (Ham 1963).

circumstances it is difficult to unequivocally recommend the use of Ham's F10 for culture of human embryos in vitro.

4.3.2 Simple Balanced Salt Solutions

The majority of IVF clinics use relatively simple balanced salt solutions for egg handling and insemination and culture of embryos. Probably the most widely used are Earle's Solution and Whittingham's T6 (Table 2). Earle's Solution needs supplementation with 11 mg/l Na pyruvate, 100 U/ml penicillin G and 10% to 15% heat inactivated serum. Earle's Balanced Salt Solution is available commercially as single strength or concentrated solution. T6 is normally prepared in the laboratory from highly purified chemicals and is also supplemented with 10%–15% human serum, although it can be used for both insemination and culture without any protein supplementation (Caro and Trounson, 1986). Another formulation, known as HTF (Human Tubal Fluid), is used by some clinics following the initial report by Quinn et al. (1985) of increased pregnancy rate compared with T6. However, in a controlled trial reported by Cummins et al. (1986a) no difference was found in IVF pregnancy rate when using HFT or T6.

These culture media (Earle's, T6 and HTF) contain high levels of bicarbonate

Table 4.2 Composition of simple media in use for human IVF

Ingredient	Earle's Balanced Salt Solution mg/l	Whittingham's T6 mg/l	Quinn's Human Tubal Fluid mg/l
NaCl	6800	5719	5939
KCl	400	106	350
NaHCO$_3$	2200	2101	2101
MgSO$_4$	100	—	49 (.7H$_2$O)
CaCl$_2$.2H$_2$O	265	262	300
Na$_2$HPO$_4$	125	51	—
KH$_2$PO$_4$	—	—	50
Glucose	1000	1000	500
Phenol red	11	10	10
Na pyruvate	—	52	36
Na lactate	—	4.65 ml/l[b]	2399
MgCl$_2$.6H$_2$O	—	96	—
Penicillin G	—	60	100 U/ml
Streptomycin SO$_4$	—	50	50
pH	7.4±0.2	7.4	[a]
H$_2$O (mosmol/kg)	275±5%	280	[a]

[a] Not given (Quinn et al. 1985).
[b] As 60% syrup.

which needs to be buffered with 5% CO_2 to prevent alkaline pH change. For egg handling, follicle flushing or other activities under normal atmospheric conditions culture media which contain a phosphate buffer or HEPES organic buffer should be used. The use of culture media which are not adequately buffered can seriously reduce the viability of eggs and embryos.

4.3.3 Serum Supplementation

The addition of human serum to culture medium is normal. Serum needs to be carefully treated. Blood should be collected in sterile non-toxic syringes, allowed to clot and centrifuged to separate the serum within a few hours of collection. The serum is then sterilized by filtration if necessary, heat inactivated in a 60 °C waterbath for 30 minutes and stored at 4 °C until required.

Filters should always be rinsed with pure water or culture medium before use and they should be of the type which do not contain wetting agents or detergent. Blood is normally taken from the patient within a few days of egg collection. The serum should be used only for the patient that it was collected from. Pooled serum should not be used because of the very serious possibility of transferring infection such as hepatitis between patients at the time of embryo replacement. It is not essential to use serum for insemination or embryo culture (Caro and Trounson 1986). Human serum can have inhibiting effects on mouse embryo development (Caro and Trounson 1984; Shirley et al. 1985) but this property of individual serum samples is not related to the patient's capacity to become pregnant by IVF (Shirley et al. 1987). The presence of protein in culture media makes handling of embryos easier and an absence of protein can result in adherence of embryos to plastic and glass surfaces. Early cleavage stage embryos metabolize very little protein (Pemble and Kaye 1986), so the protein component of serum is unlikely to have a significant role in embryo nutrition. The complex medium B3 contains human serum albumin instead of serum. Serum albumin varies considerably and at high concentrations some preparations can be toxic for mouse embryo development in vitro (Caro and Trounson 1984).

4.3.4 Physiological Fluids

It is possible that most culture media presently in use for human IVF could be considered more as diluted serum than optimal growth media. It is of interest that mouse and human eggs will fertilize and develop into embryos in human amniotic fluid (Gianaroli et al. 1986). The initial pregnancy success rate with amniotic fluid appeared to be very encouraging but subsequent multi-centre trials (L. Gianaroli and A. Trounson, unpublished data) do not show any significant increase in pregnancy rate above that obtained with T6.

Amniotic fluid is usually obtained from amniocentesis at 16–20 weeks' gestation and is used without supplementation (except for antibiotics) after heat inactivation at 60 °C for 45 minutes. Amniotic fluid contains many growth factors and other substances and is substantially different to serum. It is a very reliable medium for embryo culture but the failure to significantly increase embryo viability is disappointing. There is interest in the role of growth factors in early embryonic development but the few studies to date involving early cleavage stage mouse embryos have not shown any significant benefit for embryo viability (Caro et al. 1987). It is unlikely that insulin directly promotes early embryo cleavage because receptors for this growth promoter do not appear until the morula stage of development (Rosenblum et al. 1986).

4.3.5 Choice of Culture Medium

There are no controlled trials which reliably demonstrate any significant difference between culture media used for human IVF. It appears that the media presently in use enable human embryos to develop to the blastocyst stage in vitro but their development is probably retarded compared with that in vivo and their viability reduced with increasing time in culture. It is of interest to note that Sauer et al. (1987) obtained blastocysts from patients by flushing their uterus 5 days after the luteinizing hormone (LH) surge. This would correspond to approximately 4 days after fertilization. Blastocysts are not usually observed in vitro until the 5th or 6th day after insemination (Mohr and Trounson 1982; Cohen et al. 1985) which indicates that, like other species, human embryo development is substantially retarded in vitro. There are many reasons for retarded development of embryos in vitro and suboptimal culture medium is likely to contribute to this. It is universally accepted that mouse embryos are severely retarded when cultured in vitro. For example, Harlow and Quinn (1982) showed that 2-cell mouse embryos cultured in vitro had 45% less cells (18 cells per embryo) at the blastocyst stage than embryos grown in vivo, but there is apparently little inclination within the research community to determine the conditions which would correct this. There is, however, increasing interest in improving culture media for human IVF because this may increase IVF success rates, but little progress has been made to date. I would conclude at the moment that the medium of choice depends on the acceptance of quality control and availability of media rather than any specific type.

The need to persevere with research to optimize culture media and conditions is highlighted by the calculations of Rogers et al. (1986) who showed that embryo viability was the single most important factor governing IVF pregnancy rate and fetal development. A factor contributing to low embryo viability would be the relatively high rate of chromosomal abnormality in human eggs obtained after superovulation and follicular aspiration (Martin et al. 1986) and consequent chromosomal defects in preimplantation embryos (Angell et al. 1983). Chromosomal abnormalities are consistently reported to be 30%–40% of eggs or embryos analysed and this must limit embryo viability severely. However, the results of gamete intrafallopian transfer (GIFT) and transfer of pronuclear eggs to the fallopian tubes (PROST) are consistently as good or better than those of IVF (Table 4.3) and this difference must be due to the reduced viability of embryos cultured in vitro. There are increasing numbers of morphological abnormalities with increasing time in culture (Mohr 1984) and an increasing incidence of cells with abnormal polyploidy with increasing time in culture (Angell et al. 1987). The design of new culture media should be aimed to reduce these abnormalities and to increase the proportion of fertilized eggs which develop to the blastocyst stage at a time corresponding to that expected in vivo (4th day after insemination; Sauer et al. 1987).

Table 4.3. Pregnancy success rate for IVF, GIFT and PROST, January–March 1988 at Monash University

Procedure	No. of egg collections	No. of patient's transferred eggs or embryos	No. of pregnancies	Pregnancy success rate (%)
IVF	154	130	25	19
PROST	39	27	7	26
GIFT	49	48	17	35
Total	242	205	49	24

4.4 Culture Conditions and Methods

Insemination and culture of embryos may be carried out in culture tubes (Trounson et al. 1982), in droplets of culture medium under oil (Fishel and Jackson 1986) and in culture dishes or trays. There are advantages and disadvantages of the different methods. Culture in small tubes which are capped saves on space, maintains good pH and humidity control and the eggs and sperm are concentrated at the base of the tube. It is difficult to visualize the eggs and embryos clearly unless they are removed from the tube and pipetting them is a little more difficult. Culturing under paraffin oil maintains humidity, pH and temperature very well but oil can contaminate the laboratory, other solutions and be transferred to the patient at the time of embryo replacement. Paraffin oil can also be very toxic and care must be taken to screen batches of oil for use in culture. Most laboratories are moving to plastic culture trays or four-well dishes.

Sufficient volume is required to ensure that evaporation of medium does not cause change in the osmolarity. These culture trays have a lid which usually reduces evaporation during incubation to a minimum. The visualization and handling of eggs and embryos in such culture trays is easy. Care is required to ensure that pH, temperature and humidity are maintained during incubation and when handling the eggs and embryos.

Cultures are carried out at 37–37.5 °C under 5% CO_2 in air. It was considered preferable to culture mouse embryos under reduced oxygen (5% O_2), but there is little evidence that reduced oxygen concentrations benefit embryo development or viability in any species at the present time. There is one recent report (Carney and Bavister 1987) that the culture of 8-cell hamster embryos under 10% CO_2 gives better development to blastocysts than culture under 5% CO_2. This observation deserves further study in the mouse and human. All media should be equilibrated with CO_2 prior to use in order to control pH. This may be done by gassing medium or allowing the medium to equilibrate in a CO_2 incubator overnight.

Culture media containing pyruvate and antibiotics have a limited shelf-life even at 4 °C. It is recommended that such media should be prepared weekly from stock solutions or made complete each week. Mouse embryos synthesize pyruvate rather than glucose during early cleavage development (Gardner and Leese 1986) and the maintenance of pyruvate is probably essential in the early stages of human embryo development. Commercial media which contain pyruvate may require resupplementation and this should be determined after assay for the concentration of pyruvate in media each time it is obtained. Media which do not contain pyruvate need to be supplemented (e.g. Earle's Solution).

4.5   Evaluation of Eggs

Determination of egg quality is the single most difficult task in human IVF. It is probable that eggs from atretic follicles can be identified by the dark and gritty granulosa and that eggs from follicles which have not responded to the mid-cycle LH surge or human chorionic gonadotrophin (hGC) injection can be identified because the cumulus cells have not dispersed, the egg being surrounded by tightly packed granulosa cells. It is also possible that by using inverted microscopy the first polar body may be identified. However, this usually requires that the egg be spread on the surface of the culture dish so that the cumulus and corona radiata cells flatten away from the egg. This is usually done by placing the egg in very little culture medium and tipping the dish on an angle. This procedure is not recommended by most embryologists because of the potential damage to the egg. Studies in our own laboratory, in which we used hyaluronidase to remove the cumulus, showed that we could not predict whether an egg had extruded the first polar body or not from the degree of cumulus expansion. Johnston et al. (1987) reported that 29% of eggs with completely expanded cumuli were meiotically immature (were either at the germinal vesicle stage or at metaphase I). However, more eggs (84%) from large follicles (more than 4.5 ml follicular fluid) were mature (at metaphase II) than eggs from smaller follicles (62%).

There is no other criterion for selecting a viable oocyte at the time of collection. Even retrospective analysis of follicular fluid has yielded no reliable marker of egg viability which could be used prospectively to determine the eggs of choice to fertilize and replace in utero. Under the present circumstances the selection of eggs to use in GIFT will be more or less a random selection of those recovered from the follicles. Those used for PROST and IVF will be those which have two pronuclei and those which are developing at the expected rate in vitro respectively.

4.6 Insemination of Eggs

Motile sperm free of seminal plasma are normally added to eggs at concentrations around 10 000–500 000 sperm per ml. The normal concentration is around 50 000 sperm per ml. While it should be possible to reduce the number of sperm used for insemination there are few reports of this being attempted. One way in which the number of sperm may be reduced is to confine the volume used for insemination. In a novel approach, van der Ven et al. (1987) fertilized eggs in 5–10 μl of medium in microcapillary tubes containing 500–4000 sperm per egg (equivalent to 100 000–400 000 sperm per ml). Fertilization rates were 71%, 86%, 60% and 50% for 4000, 2000, 1000 and 500 sperm respectively. It is also apparent that less sperm are required for fertilization in small cryotubes which are placed in the patient's vagina instead of the laboratory incubator; this raises the possibility that the shaking or movement which occurs in vivo may increase the chance of fertilization. It is also of interest to note that concentrations of sperm as low as 100 per egg will fertilize zona denuded human eggs (C. Holden, R. Hyne and A. Trounson, unpublished data). This has led to the proposal that if a hole is made in the zona pellucida, by using acid from a micropipette (zona drilling) or a fine needle to crack the zona, fertilization rate may be elevated with low concentrations of sperm, particularly from male factor patients who produce few sperm. However, the human egg has no vitelline block to polyspermy and the likely outcome of these techniques is either no fertilization or polyspermy.

Increasing sperm concentrations to too high a level is likely to increase the rate of polyspermic fertilization (Wolf et al. 1984; Englert et al. 1986). This can be visualized as multiple pronuclei (more than two pronuclei). At the present time there are no sperm stimulants which have either allowed a reduction in sperm concentration from men with normal semen profiles or produced an increased fertilization rate in couples with male factor infertility.

4.7 Microfertilization Techniques

Human eggs may be fertilized by injection of single sperm under the zona pellucida using micromanipulation (Laws-King et al. 1987). This procedure involves holding the egg on a suction pipette (Fig. 4.1) after first removing the cumulus cells using hyaluronidase (Mahadevan and Trounson 1985). Sperm are incubated overnight in a medium in which calcium is replaced by strontium and then exposed to calcium briefly (Mortimer et al. 1986) before isolating individual sperm and injecting them under the zona using a finely drawn and sharpened micropipette (Fig. 4.1). Unless sperm are treated in this way, which increases the proportion of capacitated sperm, few eggs will fertilize when single sperm are injected under the zona (Metka et al. 1985; Laws-King et al. 1987). When using normal methods of sperm preparation it is necessary to inject large numbers of sperm under the zona to obtain fertilization (Lassalle et al. 1987) thus risking a substantial increase in polyspermic fertilization. This method has not been used successfully for clinical treatment of male factor infertility as yet. In our own laboratory further research on this technique has been prevented by legislation (Medical Procedures Infertility Act of Victoria) because we considered it necessary, before proceeding with clinical trials, to analyse the chromosome normality of pronuclear eggs arising from the injection of morphologically abnormal or immotile sperm from men with severe male factor infertility.

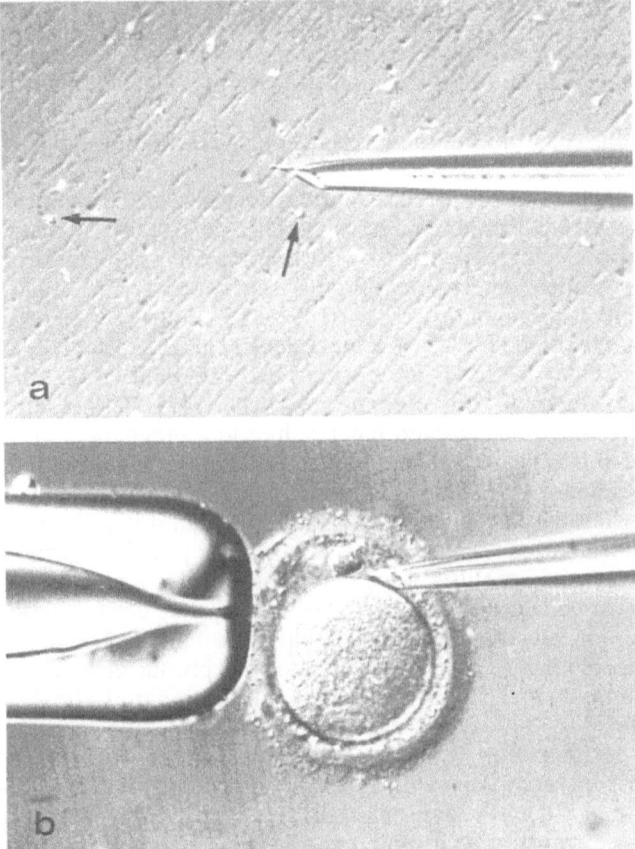

Fig. 4.1. Microfertilization technique. **a** Single sperm (*arrows*) are drawn into the sharpened micropipette and **b** injected under the zona of the egg held stationary on a suction pipette. (Reproduced with the permission of the authors and the editor from Laws-King et al. 1987.)

It has been shown in our laboratory (Mann 1988) that single mouse sperm injected into mouse eggs results in about 30% of the eggs fertilizing. These fertilized eggs develop to normal fetuses and offspring. The eggs were fertilized by sperm of normal male mice but the results do show that the selection of single sperm and micromanipulation has no effect on the normality of offspring. However, these studies do not address the possible outcome of using sperm from low quality semen. It was of interest to note in the study reported by Laws-King et al. (1987) that immotile sperm with coiled tails and twin tails are capable of fertilizing human eggs when placed under the zona pellucida.

4.8   Evaluation of the Fertilization Process

Eggs are normally examined for the presence of two distinct pronuclei (Trounson et al. 1982; see Fig. 4.2), 12–20 hours after insemination. This requires the careful dissection of the contracted cumulus cells from around the egg with fine needles (see Fishel and Jackson 1986) or with finely drawn glass pipettes. When using the latter care is required that removal of the cumulus cells is not done with pipettes which are too fine. Several different sized pipettes may be needed to achieve removal of all the cumulus cells without damage to the egg cell membrane or to the zona pellucida.

It is important to establish the presence of two pronuclei for several reasons. It has been shown that delayed fertilization and reinsemination of eggs which do not have any pronuclei and a single polar body by 20 hours after insemination is associated with severely reduced embryo viability (Trounson and Webb 1984). However, delayed insemination of mature eggs for 19 and 33 hours (Fishel et al. 1984) and immature eggs incubated for 24–30 hours (Veek et al. 1983; Boldt et al. 1987) has resulted in pregnancy. It has been reported by Boldt et al. (1987) that reinsemination of eggs which do not contain pronuclei 14–18 hours after insemination increases fertilization rate and has resulted in a pregnancy, but it was not certain whether this was a result of delayed fertilization or reinsemination. Even though it is claimed that some eggs which delay at the first cleavage develop more rapidly when they do begin cleavage (Fishel 1986) it is doubtful whether such isolated observations can be taken as a general principle because there is a certain minimum time required for DNA synthesis between cleavage divisions. One of the most concerning aspects of delayed pronuclear formation after insemination is the very substantial increase in chromosomal abnormalities. Plachot et al. (1988) reported that 87% of eggs which formed pronuclei later than 17–20 hours after insemination had chromosome anomalies, compared with 29% of eggs which had pronuclei at 17–20 hours. Of these chromosome abnormalities in eggs with delayed fertilization 30% were chromosomal mosaics in the subsequent cleavage divisions compared with 11% for eggs with pronuclei at 17–20 hours after insemination. Under these circumstances, eggs which have delayed fertilization should not be transferred to patients and it is recommended that these eggs be discarded or used for research.

Eggs with multiple pronuclei should also be discarded or used in research. Multiple pronuclei (more than two pronuclei) usually arise as a result of polyspermy (Sathananthan and Trounson 1985). Kola et al. (1987) showed that eggs with three pronuclei usually (62%) cleave directly to 3 cells with variable numbers of chromosomes approximating diploidy. These mosaic cleavage stage embryos will continue cleavage but this condition is lethal. Some tripronuclear eggs (14%) extrude a full complement of chromosomes in a small karyoplast and cleave to 2 cells. These embryos are diploid but it is not known whether the chromosomes which are retained derive from the egg and a sperm or are androgenetic with two sets of paternal (sperm) chromosomes. Some eggs (24%) also cleave to 2 cells and have a triploid complement of chromosomes. Triploidy usually causes death of the embryo or fetus but a few babies are born with multiple abnormalities and die shortly after birth. Fishel (1986) reported that 16% (4 of 25 tripronuclear eggs) developed to blastocysts in vitro but the chromosomal status of the blastocysts was not determined. Triploid or androgenetic embryos contribute to trophoblastic disease such as the hydatidiform mole and chorionic tumours. Under these circumstances embryos which derive from multiple pronuclei should not be replaced in utero and this necessitates that eggs be carefully examined at the pronuclear stage 12–20 hours after insemination.

4.9   Evaluation of Embryos

Much has been written about the evaluation of embryos and the general agreement is that embryos which divide evenly (Fig. 4.2), regularly and rapidly are the embryos with the highest viability or capacity for development to term when replaced in utero. However, many examples have been noted where retarded and unevenly cleaved embryos develop to term so there are no absolute criteria available at present to determine which embryos are viable and which are not. Consequently it is usual that the more advanced and evenly cleaved embryos of any cohort are usually replaced in utero.

The most detailed study of embryo cleavage rate and association with pregnancy has been reported by Cummins et al. (1986b). They showed the coupling of a subjective score (1–4) of embryo quality based on the symmetry of cleavage, evenness of the cytoplasm and presence or absence of anucleate fragments, together with a rating of their cleavage based on the ratio between the observed cleavage stage and expected cleavage stage, gave a good guide to expected pregnancy. Both the subjective score and the rating for cleavage stage were significantly correlated to each other and to pregnancy. The overall result of these analyses demonstrated that the rapidly dividing embryos which were not scored as subjectively of poor quality (lowest rating) were the embryos most likely to contribute to pregnancy. They were able to confirm their results in 33 single embryo transfers which resulted in pregnancy; the one low score for cleavage rate resulted in miscarriage. The only unusual observation in this study was that embryos which were very advanced relative to the expected cleavage stage were not more likely to contribute to pregnancy than the general population of embryos. Examining their data it appears that providing the advanced embryos were not of poor quality their contributions to pregnancy were similar to that for rapidly dividing embryos (above the expected cleavage stage). The final conclu-

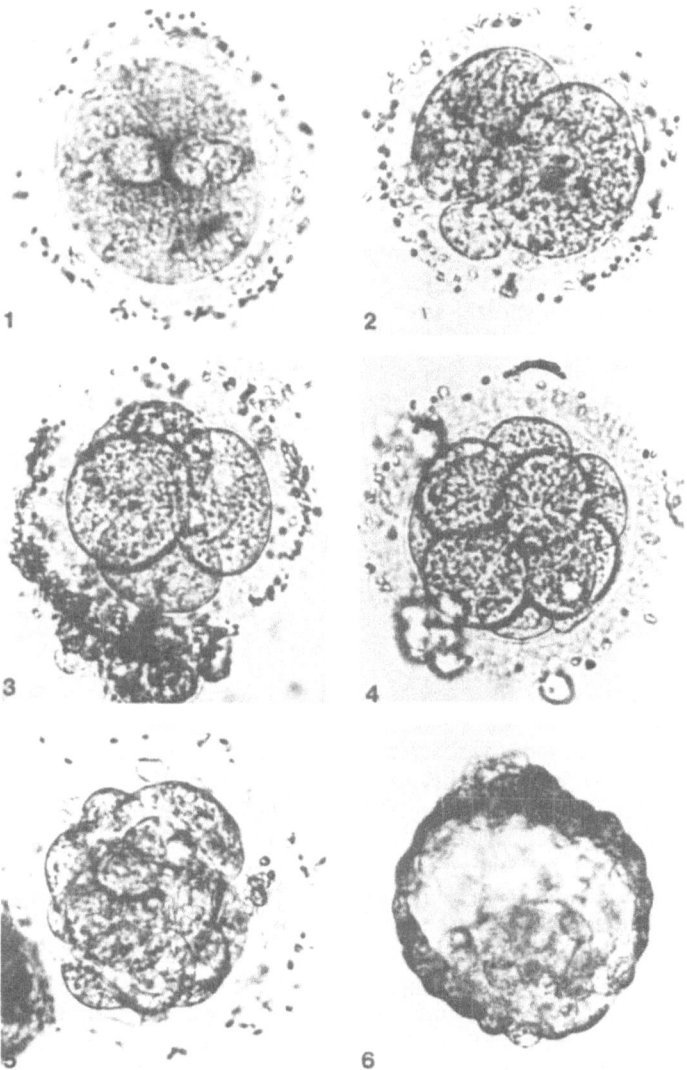

Fig. 4.2.   Cleavage stage human pre-implantation embryos. 1, a pronuclear egg; 2, a 2-cell embryo; 3, a 4-cell embryo; 4, an 8-cell embryo; 5, a morula; 6, a hatched blastocyst. (Reproduced with the permission of the authors and Editor. From Trounson et al. 1982.)

sion that can be drawn from this study is that embryos assessed as poor quality have markedly reduced viability and those which cleave rapidly to the expected stage of development have increased viability. This supports earlier observations which indicated that the more rapidly dividing embryos are more likely to contribute to pregnancy (Trounson et al. 1982). However, Testart (1986) was unable to associate cleavage stage and pregnancy with the simple data he used, but Puissant et al. (1987) found that embryos, subjectively scored as good quality based on the degree of anucleate fragmentation and cleavage rate to 4 cells, were more often associated with pregnancy and with multiple pregnancy.

Examples of normal and abnormal features of cleaving embryos and blasto-cysts have been given in many publications and have been best dealt with by Edwards et al. (1981), Mohr et al. (1983), Mohr (1984), Lopata et al. (1983), Mohr and Trounson (1984), Sathananthan (1984), Trounson and Sathananthan (1984), Sathananthan et al. (1985) and Fishel (1986). While these examples of morphology viewed under dissecting microscopy and electron microscopy are helpful in evaluating embryos there is a need to develop more noninvasive tests of embryonic normality. It is possible that by using quantitative fluorescence microscopy, the uptake of pyruvate and glucose by single embryos may give an indication of human embryo viability (Leese et al. 1986; Leese 1987). However, these tests will not indicate genetic normality. It has been calculated that 20%–50% of human eggs and cleavage stage embryos have chromosomal anomalies (Angell et al. 1983, 1986, 1987; Martin et al. 1986; Plachot et al. 1986, 1988; Warmsby et al. 1987). Identification of these defects will probably require the development of cell sampling (embryo biopsy) techniques (Wilton and Trounson 1988) or major alterations to superovulation and IVF techniques to reduce their occurrence. This should be a priority of research in IVF.

4.10 Conclusions

There appears to be little difference in fertilization rate and embryo development between the various media presently in use for human IVF. It is, however, important to institute strict quality control measures in the culture laboratory to maintain consistent success in IVF. New materials should be tested before they are introduced, using mouse embryo or cell culture test systems, and culture media regularly tested for their suitability for embryo culture.

There is no absolute selection criterion available for determining egg and embryo viability. If immature eggs are identified they may be cultured for 20–24 hours before insemination but viability of such eggs is likely to be reduced. Eggs which do not have pronuclei by 17–20 hours are likely to have increased chromosomal anomalies. These eggs and those with multiple pronuclei should be discarded and not reinseminated or replaced in the patients.

Studies on human eggs and embryos reveal relatively high rates of chromoso-mal anomalies. Strategies need to be developed to reduce this if possible, including an examination of chromosomal normality of naturally ovulated eggs. There is also a need to improve present culture conditions and media to increase the rate of embryo cleavage and development in vitro. This is likely to increase embryo viability because of the association of pregnancy in IVF with the more rapidly dividing embryos replaced in utero. Fragmented and poor quality embryos, judged subjectively, also have reduced viability. These problems may derive from incomplete or abnormal egg maturation, or from suboptimal culture conditions.

References

Ackerman SB, Swanson RJ, Stokes GK, Veeck LL (1984) Culture of mouse preimplantation embryos as a quality control assay for human in vitro fertilization. Gamete Res 9:145–152

Ackerman SB, Stokes GL, Swanson RJ, Taylor SP, Fenwick L (1985) Toxicity testing for human in vitro fertilization programs. J In Vitro Fert Embryo Transfer 2:132–137

Angell RR, Aitken RJ, Van Look PFA, Lumsden MA, Templeton AA (1983) Chromosome abnormalities in human embryos in in vitro fertilization. Nature 303:336

Angell RR, Templeton AA, Aitken RJ (1986) Chromosome studies in human in vitro fertilization. Hum Genet 72:333–339

Angell RR, Sumner AT, West JD, Thatcher SS, Glasier AF, Baird DT (1987) Post-fertilization polyploidy in human preimplantation embryos fertilized in vitro. Human Reprod 2:721–727

Biggers JD, Whitten WK, Whittingham DG (1971) The culture of mouse embryos in vitro. In: Daniel JC (ed) Methods in mammalian embryology. WH Freeman, San Francisco, pp 86–116

Boldt J, Howe AM, Butler WJ, McDonough PG, Padilla SL (1987) The value of oocyte reinsemination in human in vitro fertilization. Fertil Steril 48:617–623

Carney EW, Bavister BD (1987) Regulation of hamster embryo development in vitro by carbon dioxide. Biol Reprod 36:1155–1163

Caro CM, Trounson A (1984) The effect of protein on preimplantation mouse embryo development in vitro. J In Vitro Fert Embryo Transfer 1:183–187

Caro CM, Trounson A (1986) Successful fertilization, embryo development, and pregnancy in human in vitro fertilization (IVF) using a chemically defined culture medium containing no protein. J In Vitro Fert Embryo Transfer 3:215–217

Caro CM, Trounson A, Kirby C (1987) Effect of growth factors in culture medium on the rate of mouse development and viability in vitro. J In Vitro Fert Embryo Transfer 4:265–268

Cohen J, Simons RF, Edwards RG, Fehilly CB, Fishel SB (1985) Pregnancies following the frozen storage of expanding human blastocysts. J In Vitro Fert Embryo Transfer 2:59–64

Cummins JM, Breen TM, Fuller SM et al. (1986a) Comparison of two media in a human in vitro fertilization program: lack of significant differences in pregnancy rate. J In Vitro Fert Embryo Transfer 3:326–329

Cummins JM, Breen TM, Harrison KL, Shaw JM, Wilson LM, Hennessey JF (1986b) A formula for scoring human embryo growth rates in in vitro fertilization: its value in predicting pregnancy and in comparison with visual estimates of embryo quality. J In Vitro Fert Embryo Transfer 3:284–295

Edwards RG, Purdy JM, Steptoe PC, Walters DE (1981) The growth of human preimplantation embryos in vitro. Am J Obstet Gynecol 141:408–416

Englert Y, Puissant F, Camus M, Degueldre M, Leroy F (1986) Factors leading to tripronucleate eggs during human in vitro fertilization. Human Reprod 1:117–119

Fishel S (1986) Growth of the human conceptus in vitro. In: Fishel S, Symonds EM (eds) In vitro fertilisation: past, present and future. IRL Press, Oxford, pp 107–126

Fishel S, Jackson P (1986) Preparation for human in vitro fertilization in the laboratory. In: Fishel S, Symonds EM (eds) In vitro fertilisation: past, present and future. IRL Press, Oxford, pp. 77–87

Fishel SB, Edwards RG, Purdy JM (1984) Births after a prolonged delay between oocyte recovery and fertilization in vitro. Gamete Res 9:175–181

Fukuda A, Noda Y, Tsukui S, Matsumoto H, Yano J, Mori T (1987) Influence of water quality on in vitro fertilization and embryo development for the mouse. J In Vitro Fert Embryo Transfer 4:40–45

Gardner DK, Leese HJ (1986) Non-invasive measurement of nutrient uptake by single cultured preimplantation mouse embryos. Human Reprod 1:25–27

Gianaroli L, Seracchioli R, Ferraretti AP, Trounson A, Flamigni C, Bovicelli L (1986) The successful use of human amniotic fluid for mouse embryo culture and human in vitro fertilization, embryo culture and embryo transfer. Fertil Steril 46:907–913

Ham RG (1963) An improved nutrient solution for diploid Chinese hamster and human cell lines Exp Cell Res 29:515–526

Harlow GM, Quinn P (1982) Development of preimplantation mouse embryos in vivo and in vitro. Aust J Biol Sci 35:187–193

Johnston I, Lopata A, Pepperell RJ, Trounson A, Wood C (1987) The use of in vitro fertilization in the infertile couple. In: Pepperell RJ, Hudson B, Wood C (eds) The infertile couple. Churchill Livingstone, Edinburgh, pp 263–312

Kola I, Trounson AO, Dawson G, Rogers P (1987) Tripronuclear human oocytes: altered cleavage patterns and subsequent karyotypic analysis of embryos. Biol Reprod 37:395–401

Lassalle B, Courtot AM, Testart J (1987) In vitro fertilization of hamster and human oocytes by microinjection of human sperm. Gamete Res 16:69–78

Laws-King A, Trounson A, Sathananthan H, Kola I (1987) Fertilization of human oocytes by microinjection of a single spermatozoon under the zona pellucida. Fertil Steril 48:637–642

Leese HJ (1987) Non-invasive methods of assessing embryos. Human Reprod 2:435–438

Leese HJ, Hooper MAK, Edwards RG, Ashwood-Smith MJ (1986) Uptake of pyruvate by early human embryos determined by a non-invasive technique. Human Reprod 1:181–182

Lopata A, Kohlman D, Johnston I (1983) The fine structure of normal and abnormal human embryos developed in culture. In: Beier HM, Lindner HR (eds) Fertilization of the human egg in vitro. Springer-Verlag, Berlin Heidelberg New York, pp 189–210

Loutradis D, John D, Kiessling AA (1987) Hypoxanthine causes a 2-cell block in random-bred mouse embryos. Biol Reprod 37:311–316

McMaster R, Yanagimachi R, Lopata A (1978) Penetration of human eggs by human spermatozoa in vitro. Biol Reprod 19:212–216

Mahadevan M, Baker G (1984) Assessment and preparation of semen for in vitro fertilization. In: Wood C, Trounson A (eds) Clinical in vitro fertilization. Springer-Verlag, Berlin Heidelberg New York, pp 83–98

Mahadevan MM, Trounson AO (1985) Removal of the cumulus oophorus from the human oocyte for in vitro fertilization. Fertil Steril 43:263–267

Mann JR (1988) Full term development of mouse eggs fertilized by a spermatozoon microinjected under the zona pellucida. Biol Reprod 38:1077–1083

Martin RH, Mahadevan MM, Taylor PJ et al. (1986) Chromosomal analysis of unfertilized human oocytes. J Reprod Fertil 78:663–678

Menezo Y (1976) Milieu synthetique pour la survie et la maturation des gametes et pour la culture de l'oeuf feconde. C R Acad Sci III 282: 1967–1970

Menezo Y, Testart J, Perrone D (1984) Serum is not necessary in human in vitro fertilization, early embryo culture, and transfer. Fertil Steril 42:750–755

Metka M, Haromy T, Huber J, Schurz B (1985) Artificial insemination using a micromanipulator. Fertilität 1:41–44

Mohr LR (1984) Assessment of human embryos. In: Trounson A, Wood C (eds) In vitro fertilization and embryo transfer. Churchill Livingstone, Edinburgh, pp 159–171

Mohr LR, Trounson AO (1982) Comparative ultrastructure of the hatched human, mouse and bovine blastocysts. J Reprod Fertil 66:499–504

Mohr L, Trounson A. (1984) In vitro fertilization and embryo growth. In: Wood C, Trounson A (eds) Clinical in vitro fertilization. Springer-Verlag, Berlin Heidelberg New York, pp 99–116

Mohr LR, Trounson AO, Leeton JF, Wood C (1983) Evaluation of normal and abnormal human embryo development during procedures in vitro. In: Beier HM, Lidner HR (eds) Fertilization of the human egg in vitro. Springer-Verlag, Berlin Heidelberg New York, pp 169–188

Mortimer D, Curtis EF, Dravland JE (1986) The use of strontium-substituted media for capacitating human spermatozoa: an improved sperm preparation method for the zona-free hamster egg penetration test. Fertil Steril 46:97–103

Parinaud J, Reme J-M, Monrozies X, Favrin S, Sarramon M-F, Pontonnier G (1987) Mouse system quality control is necessary before the use of new material for in vitro fertilization and embryo transfer. J In Vitro Fert Embryo Transfer 4:56–58

Pemble LB, Kaye PL (1986) Whole protein uptake and metabolism by mouse blastocysts. J Reprod Fertil 78:149–157

Plachot M, Junca AM, Mandelbaum J, de Grouchy J, Salat-Baroux J, Cohen J (1986) Chromosome investigations in early life. I. Human oocytes recovered in an IVF program. Human Reprod 1:547–551

Plachot M, de Grouchy J, Junca A-M, Mandelbaum J, Salat-Baroux J, Cohen J (1988) Chromosome analysis of human oocytes and embryos: does delayed fertilization increase chromosome imbalance? Human Reprod 3:125–127

Puissant F, Rysselberge MV, Barlow P, Deweze J, Leroy F (1987) Embryo scoring as a prognostic tool in IVF treatment. Human Reprod 2:705–708

Quinn P, Kerin JF, Warnes GM (1985) Improved pregnancy rate in human in vitro fertilization with the use of a medium based on the composition of human tubal fluid. Fertil Steril 44:493–498

Ray BD, McDermott A, Wardle PG et al. (1987) In vitro fertilization: fertilization failure due to toxic catheters. J In Vitro Fert Embryo Transfer 4:58–61

Rogers PAW, Milne BJ, Trounson AO (1986) A model to show human uterine receptivity and embryo viability following ovarian stimulation for in vitro fertilization J In Vitro Fert Embryo Transfer 3:93–98

Rosenblum IY, Mattson BA, Heyner S (1986) Stage-specific insulin binding in mouse preimplantation embryos. Dev Biol 116:261–263

Sathananthan AH (1984) Ultrastructural morphology of fertilization and early cleavage in the human. In: Trounson A, Wood C (eds) In vitro fertilization and embryo transfer. Churchill Livingstone, Edinburgh, pp 131–171

Sathananthan AH, Trounson AO (1985) The human pronuclear ovum: fine structure of monospermic and polyspermic fertilization in vitro. Gamete Res 12:385–398

Sathananthan AH, Trounson AO, Wood C (1985) Ultrastructural atlas of human fertilization and embryonic development. Praeger, Philadelphia

Sauer MV, Bustillo M, Rodi IA, Gorrill MJ, Buster JE (1987) In vivo blastocyst production and ovum yield among fertile women. Human Reprod 2:701–703

Shirley B, Wortham JWE Jr, Witmyer J, Condon-Mahony M, Fort G (1985) Effects of human serum and plasma on development of mouse embryos in culture media. Fertil Steril 43:129–134

Shirley B, Wortham JWE Jr, Peoples D, White S, Condon-Mahony M (1987) Inhibition of embryo development by some maternal sera. J In Vitro Fert Embryo Transfer 4:93–97

Silverman IH, Cook CL, Sanfilippo JS, Schultz GS, Yassman MA, Hilton FK (1987) Ham's F-10 constituted with tap water supports mouse conceptus development in vitro. J In Vitro Fert Embryo Transfer 4:185–187

Testart J (1986) Cleavage stage of human embryos two days after fertilization in vitro and their developmental ability after transfer into the uterus. Human Reprod 1:29–31

Trounson AO, Sathananthan AH (1984) The application of electron microscopy in the evaluation of 2–4 cell human embryos cultured in vitro for embryo transfer. J In Vitro Fert Embryo Transfer 1:153–165

Trounson A, Webb J (1984) Fertilization of human oocytes following reinsemination in vitro. Fertil Steril 41:816–819

Trounson AO, Mohr LR, Wood C, Leeton JF (1982) Effect of delayed insemination in in vitro fertilization, culture and transfer of human embryos. J Reprod Fert 64:285–294

van der Ven HH, Hoebbel K, Al-Hasani S, Diedrich K, Krebs D (1987) Befruchtung menschlicher Eizellen in Kapillarröhrehen mit sehr geringen Spermatozoenzahlen. Geburtshilfe Frauenheilkd 47:630–635

Veeck LL, Wortham JWE, Witmyer J (1983) Maturation and fertilization of morphologically immature human oocytes in a program of in vitro fertilization. Fertil Steril 39:594–602

Warmsby H, Fredga K, Leidholm P (1987) Chromosome analysis of human oocytes recovered from preovulatory follicles in stimulated cycles. N Engl J Med 316:121–124

Whittingham DG (1971) Culture of mouse ova. J Reprod Fertil [Suppl] 14:7–21

Wilton LJ, Trounson AO (1988) Biopsy of pre-implantation mouse embryos: development of micromanipulated embryos and proliferation of single blastomeres in vitro. Biol Reprod (in press)

Wolf DP, Byrd W, Dandekar P, Quigley MM (1984) Sperm concentration and the fertilization of human eggs in vitro. Biol Reprod 31:837–848

Wood C, Trounson A (1982) In vitro fertilization and embryo transfer. In: Bonnar J (ed) Recent advances in obstetrics and gynaecology. Churchill Livingstone, Edinburgh, pp 259–282

Yanagimachi R (1984) Zona-free hamster eggs: their use in assessing fertilizing capacity and examining chromosomes of human spermatozoa. Gamete Res 10:187–232

5 Results from In Vitro Fertilization

H. W. Jones Jr and P. A. W. Rogers

5.1 The Evaluation of Results

H. W. Jones Jr

The results of a programme of in vitro fertilization (IVF) would seem to be simple enough to state: as a numerator one has the number of pregnancies, and as denominator the number of attempts. However, there are problems in identifying precisely the numbers to be included in the numerator and denominator.

5.1.1 Numerator Problems

It is not easy to arrive at a satisfactory numerator to express the pregnancy rate for an IVF programme; this is because, specifically, the definition of a pregnancy is not easy. In a non-medical setting the pronouncement of pregnancy seems relatively simple – a missed menstrual period plus a positive pregnancy test.

It is generally stated that the expectancy of a miscarriage is about 15% of all pregnancies in a non-medical setting. Careful study has shown that this percentage is most probably nearer 20% (French and Biermann 1962). However in one study of women who discontinued contraception with the intention of achieving pregnancy, and where they were monitored with a very sensitive test for beta-human chorionic gonadotrophin (β-hCG), it was shown that 61.9% of concepti were lost prior to 12 weeks. Most of these losses occurred in association with a menstrual period and without the mother's knowledge (Edmonds et al. 1982). Thus, the incidence of pregnancy is directly related to the zeal with which those exposed to pregnancy are monitored, especially by tests for β-hCG. This is a special problem for IVF programmes. For example, Lenton and colleagues studied material from the IVF programme in Manchester and demonstrated that there were a number of small rises in β-hCG, sometimes delayed in patients who exhibited no clinical signs of pregnancy (Lenton et al. 1987). Furthermore, Liu and colleagues, in studying the material from Norfolk, found that with a very sensitive test they were able to demonstrate transient rises in β-hCG, together with rises in oestradiol (E_2) and sometimes progesterone (P_4), among 10% of patients who were considered in a routine evaluation as being non-pregnant (Liu et al. 1987). Programmes of IVF vary considerably in their definition of pregnancy; therefore, in evaluating the results from a programme, one must obviously have a clear statement of the definition. For example, in the Norfolk programme, the administration of 10 000 IU of hCG as a luteotrophic hormone (LH) surrogate for the LH surge affords only an uncertain opportunity to pick up an elevated β-hCG, unless it is done under very careful circumstances, as in Liu's study, before the menstrual period expected after the egg harvest. It may take as long as 10–12 days for the injected hCG to clear.

Very early pregnancies (sometimes referred to as biochemical pregnancies) cannot be identified with certainty in the Norfolk programme except under very special conditions. In this connection Edmonds and colleagues (1982) showed that an elevated β-hCG from a conceptus could sometimes be found as soon as 6 days after ovulation. Therefore, it became necessary in the Norfolk programme to require that any elevated value of β-hCG obtained no earlier than day 12 after egg harvest be followed by a higher value before pregnancy was diagnosed. In practice an elevated β-hCG value on day 12 is likely to be from the conceptus, but the diagnosis of pregnancy cannot be made with any certainty on a single elevated value of β-hCG. Rising E_2 and P_4 values late in the luteal phase can be considered supportive signs of pregnancy. In fact, elevations in E_2 values after a fall of E_2 values in the luteal phase are often a much earlier sign of pregnancy than is a positive test for β-hCG.

In IVF programmes the outcome of pregnancy needs to be specified as part of the routine data and can be done in a variety of ways. In Norfolk, pregnancy outcome is classified as preclinical abortion, clinical abortion or viable pregnancy (Jones et al. 1983).

5.1.1.1 Preclinical Abortion

Preclinical abortion designates those situations in which a pregnancy, as defined above, is terminated by the onset of a menstrual period not later than 28 days after egg harvest and fertilization; i.e. the menses may be delayed no more than 14 days. It is to be noted that the adjective *preclinical* refers to the abortion and not to the pregnancy. The abortion is called preclinical because it is indistinguishable from the menstrual period. No grossly recognized tissue is passed, and no clinical action is necessary.

5.1.1.2 Clinical Abortion

The term clinical abortion refers to spontaneous termination 4 weeks after egg harvest and prior to viability. Generally, among patients who have had a clinical abortion, a dilatation and curettage needs to be performed. Thus, a clinical action has been necessary.

5.1.1.3 Viable Pregnancy

The term viable pregnancy refers to all other pregnancies. The most desirable situation – and the most meaningful numerator – would be a viable pregnancy. Most IVF programmes include in the numerator the viable pregnancies plus the clinical abortions. However, many include some or all of the preclinical abortions, and some include transient rises of β-hCG prior to an expected menstrual period. Thus, there is bound to be considerable variation from programme to programme in the percentage of so-called biochemical pregnancies and preclinical abortions included in the numerator pregnancies.

A rough index of what is included in the numerator may be obtained by a statement of the viable pregnancy rate in relation to the total pregnancy rate. This particular value also seems to vary from programme to programme, and abortion rates of up to almost 50% have sometimes been reported.

5.1.2 Denominator Problems

The denominator to express a pregnancy rate can be derived in various ways. The most comprehensive denominator would include all patients screened by history but not by actual attendance at the IVF centre. This denominator is an impracticality because record keeping may be imprecise and programmes vary in rejection rates at this point. However, the rejection rate at this stage, if known, would be a useful index.

The next most comprehensive denominator would include all patients interviewed and examined. Again, rejection and selection are important variables which are almost never stated in end result data.

The number of patients who enter stimulation for the harvesting of eggs is a useful method of reporting the denominator. The drop-out rate between entering stimulation and harvest gives a cancellation rate, which is a key index to the efficiency of oocyte recruitment. The drop-out rate, for the most part, is determined by the patient's failure to respond to the stimulation.

The number of patients who undergo embryo transfer has come into wide-spread use as the denominator and has the advantage of eliminating variables due to failed harvest, or failed fertilization. A useful index is the transfer rate, which is the number of patients having embryos transferred divided by the number of patients *harvested*.

The denominator factor can be further refined by limiting it to certain types of eggs inseminated. If only fully mature eggs are inseminated, as is customary in most programmes, the denominator tends to be smaller since those patients whose eggs are immature will be eliminated. This will tend to raise the pregnancy rate, as pregnancy expectancy from immature eggs which are matured in vitro is far less than that from fully mature eggs (Veeck 1984).

The end results from IVF programmes are difficult for the reading public to ascertain – and, indeed, sometimes difficult for those involved in a programme. Unfortunately, the results are also subject to manipulation. The reader must be well informed about the factors which constitute the numerator and the denominator before he can be confident that the end results are expressing what he wishes to know.

5.2 Results

P. A. W. Rogers

The results summarized in this chapter come from five Australian IVF programmes: the Queen Elizabeth Hospital in Adelaide (QEH), the Queensland

Fertility Group in Brisbane (QFG), the Monash/Queen Victoria/Epworth programme in Melbourne (Monash), the Royal North Shore Hospital in Sydney (RNS), and the Royal Womens' Hospital in Melbourne (RWH). The data presented cover the years 1982–1986 and are given separately for each year. Where relevant data were not kept or the information is presently unavailable a question mark (?) has been placed in the appropriate column.

5.2.1 Ovulation Induction and Oocyte Retrieval

The percentage of patients reaching oocyte retrieval once treatment for IVF has commenced varies considerably from group to group (Table 5.1). This differing drop-out rate is primarily due to differences in policy between groups as to what is an acceptable response to ovulation induction. However, the drop-out rate can also be influenced by other factors, such as the selection of particular types of patients (e.g. endocrine-abnormal or previous poor responders to ovulation induction). Unscheduled problems such as illness that may result in the patient cancelling after treatment has commenced can also add significantly to the drop-out rate. The data in Table 5.1 show that drop-out rates remain relatively constant from year to year within each group. Whether or not the drop-out criteria used by each group are effective in increasing the overall pregnancy rate is unknown; however this could be resolved by a controlled trial between two groups with significantly different drop-out criteria. More recent information from Monash (unpublished data) suggests that prospective selection of patients into groups with either a good or a poor prognosis can result in two groups with very different pregnancy rates.

Combined clomiphene citrate/human menopausal gonadotrophin (CC/hMG) has been established as the ovulation induction protocol of choice (Table 5.2). More recently the gonadotrophin releasing hormone (GnRH) agonist, buserelin, has been successfully used to suppress endogenous gonadotrophin secretion and allow high rates of follicular recruitment using exogenous gonadotrophins alone (Healy et al. 1987). While this approach to ovulation induction for IVF is still in

Table 5.1. Numbers of patients reaching oocyte retrieval following commencement of standard IVF treatment (not GIFT)

	1982	1983	1984	1985	1986	Total
QEH	103	167	255	307	360	1192
	128 (80%)	229 (73%)	344 (74%)	419 (73%)	503 (72%)	1623 (73%)
QFG	?	?	593	969	1032	2594
			620 (96%)	998 (97%)	1200 (86%)	2818 (92%)
Monash	340	518	607	734	845	3044
	418 (81%)	602 (86%)	684 (89%)	858 (86%)	1022 (83%)	3584 (85%)
RNS	173	296	482	572	526	2049
	?	?	?	?	?	?
RWH	336	401	489	491		1717
	?	?	?	?	?	?

Table 5.2. Method of ovulation induction for IVF (figures given as percentage of patients receiving each type of ovulation induction in each year)

	1982 (%)	1983 (%)	1984 (%)	1985 (%)	1986 (%)
QEH					
Clomid/hMG	42	55	91	99	95
Clomid only	58	45	7	0	0
hMG only	0	0	0	1	2
Other	0	0	2	0	3
QFG					
Clomid/hMG	—	100	100	99	95
Clomid only	—	0	0	0	0
hMG only	—	0	0	1	5
Other	—	0	0	0	0
Monash					
Clomid/hMG	78	97	97	94	90
Clomid only	17	0	0	0	0
hMG only	4	2	2	2	2
Other	1	1	1	4	8
RNS					
Clomid/hMG	10	83	86	98	100
Clomid only	90	17	1	2	0
hMG only	0	0	13	0	0
Other	0	0	0	0	0

Data from RWH unavailable.

Table 5.3. Relative use of hCG versus spontaneous LH surge in timing for oocyte retrieval (figures given in percentages for each year)

	1982 (%)	1983 (%)	1984 (%)	1985 (%)	1986 (%)
QEH					
LH	36	58	34	45	42
hCG	64	42	66	55	58
QFG					
LH	—	—	95	90	70
hCG	—	—	5	10	30
Monash					
LH	64	69	44	29	20
hCG	36	31	56	71	80
RNS					
LH	0	1	1	0	0
hCG	100	99	99	100	100

Data from RWH unavailable.

its infancy it is possible that the advantages it confers in terms of suppression of unscheduled luteinizing hormone (LH) surges and increased oocyte numbers may well make it the method of choice in the future.

Scheduling of oocyte retrieval from either a spontaneous LH surge or by hCG injection varies considerably from group to group (Table 5.3). However, neither approach appears to confer a significant advantage, other than the fact that hCG injection avoids the administrative problems that can occur with a large number of unscheduled oocyte retrievals.

Prior to 1984 all oocyte retrievals were by laparoscopy (Table 5.4). From this time on ultrasound-guided pickups were performed by some groups on a trial basis. By 1986 transvaginal ultrasound-guided follicle aspiration was becoming the technique of choice for several groups. The ability to treat women on an outpatient basis with this approach suggests that vaginal ultrasound retrievals will be the dominant method in the near future.

Table 5.4. Method of oocyte retrieval (figures given as percentages for each year.)

	1982 (%)	1983 (%)	1984 (%)	1985 (%)	1986 (%)
QEH					
Laparoscopy	100	100	86	94	63
Vaginal ultrasound	0	0	0	0	13
Abdominal ultrasound	0	0	14	5	5
GIFT	0	0	0	1	19
QFG					
Laparoscopy	—	—	100	100	89
Vaginal ultrasound	—	—	0	0	3
Abdominal ultrasound	—	—	0	0	0
GIFT	—	—	0	0	8
Monash					
Laparoscopy	100	100	100	100	18
Vaginal ultrasound	0	0	0	0	77
Abdominal ultrasound	0	0	0	0	0
GIFT	0	0	0	0	5
RNS					
Laparoscopy	100	100	86	75	19
Vaginal ultrasound	0	0	0	2	59
Abdominal ultrasound	0	0	14	23	0
GIFT	0	0	0	0	22
RWH					
Laparoscopy	100	100	100	88	65
Vaginal ultrasound	0	0	0	0	1
Abdominal ultrasound	0	0	0	0	0
GIFT	0	0	0	12	34

5.2.2   Fertilization and Embryo Transfer

The percentage of follicles that yield an oocyte falls in the range of 70%–80% for most IVF programmes over most years. With the advent of ultrasound-guided oocyte retrievals it became possible to visualize more follicles than was previously possible by laparoscopy. This was particularly the case in patients with restricted laparoscopic access due to pelvic adhesions. At Monash there was a significant drop in the follicular oocyte recovery rate from 77% to 64% with the introduction of ultrasound-guided retrievals. However, this was balanced by an increase in the average number of oocytes retrieved per patient from 4.7 in 1985 to 5.1 in 1986. This increase is undoubtedly due to the better ovarian visualization and access offered by ultrasound.

Fertilization rates in IVF will vary markedly depending primarily on the quality of the semen. The use of IVF to treat couples where the husband has subnormal semen quality has not been embraced equally by all programmes (Table 5.5). Using normal semen (count greater than 20 million/ml, motility greater than 40% abnormal forms less than 40%), fertilization rates of between 70% and 80% should be achieved with routine IVF. The prognosis for patients with subnormal semen varies considerably depending on the severity of the problem. At Monash patients with reductions in only one or two of the three parameters (count, motility and abnormal forms) tend to average about 50% fertilization rates, while those with defects in all three categories may achieve fertilization rates of less than 10% (Yates and de Kretser 1987).

Regardless of ovulation induction drop-out criteria or percentage of subnormal semen patients, between 80% and 90% of all patients having oocyte retrieval reach the embryo transfer stage of IVF (Table 5.6). However, it is well documented that pregnancy success rates correlate strongly with the number and quality of the embyros replaced at transfer (Rogers et al. 1986; Cummins et al. 1986). For this reason embryo transfer alone is not necessarily a good indicator by which to judge the success or otherwise of an IVF treatment cycle.

5.2.3 Pregnancy

Total pregnancy rate per transfer for all five groups varied between 16% and 23% in 1986 and from 12% to 18% in 1985, (Table 5.7). In general terms the total pregnancy rate per transfer has not improved significantly since 1982, suggesting that some major breakthrough in our understanding of the barriers to successful IVF will be required to improve this situation.

Pregnancy outcome for each IVF group is given in Table 5.8. Successful outcomes occurred in 64%–75% of all pregnancies, with the highest wastage being due to abortions (13%–26% of all pregnancies ended in spontaneous abortion). The ectopic pregnancy rate following IVF ranges from 2% to 5%. This rate is significantly higher than that seen following natural conception (Martinez and Trounson 1986), although these authors could find no clear reason as to why this may be so.

Further detailed analysis of pregnancies derived from Australian IVF programmes can be found in the publication of the National Perinatal Statistics Unit titled "In vitro fertilization pregnancies, Australia and New Zealand, 1979–1985". Data from this survey show that 77.6% of pregnancies reaching 20 weeks of gestation were singleton, 18.7% twins, 3.5% triplets and 0.1% quadruplets. The bulk of pregnancies occurred when the maternal age was in the 30–34 year range, and the most common duration of infertility for patients achieving pregnancy through IVF was 4–5 years. The incidence of spontaneous abortion increased from 21% in the 30–34 year age group up to 44% in the 40+ years age group. Perhaps the most significant information revealed by this major study is the increased incidence of preterm birth, low birth weight and perinatal mortality in infants resulting from IVF. Among all infants in this study 26.6% were classified as preterm (less than 37 weeks) and 34.8% were low birth weight (less

Table 5.5. Fertilization statistics for patients undertaking standard IVF

	1982	1983	1984	1985	1986	Total
OEH						
Follicles aspirated	301	698	1307	2036	2557	6899
Oocytes collected	246 (82%)	514 (74%)	1001 (77%)	1396 (69%)	1954 (76%)	5111 (74%)
Oocytes fertilized	147	366	692	953	1204	3362
with normal semen	206 (71%)	496 (74%)	932 (74%)	1213 (79%)	1590 (76%)	4437 (52%)
Oocytes fertilized	23	9	31	95	192	350
with subnormal semen	40 (58%)	18 (50%)	69 (45%)	183 (52%)	364 (53%)	674 (52%)
Monash						
Follicles aspirated	?	2177	3141	4467	6745	16530
Oocytes collected	?	1683 (77%)	2442 (78%)	3425 (77%)	4303 (64%)	11853 (72%)
Oocytes fertilized	—	453	1493	1630	2178	5301
with normal semen	?	?	2045 (73%)	2341 (70%)	3105 (70%)	7491 (71%)
Oocytes fertilized	—	?	166	322	377	865
with subnormal semen	?	?	333 (50%)	777 (41%)	638 (59%)	1748 (49%)
RNS						
Follicles aspirated	427	903	2564	2320	?	6214
Oocytes collected	291 (68%)	669 (74%)	2185 (85%)	1662 (72%)	?:	4807 (77%)
Oocytes fertilized	163	453	1564	1180		3360
with normal semen	291 (56%)	669 (68%)	2185 (72%)	1662 (71%)	?	4807 (70%)
RWH						
Follicles aspirated	1786	2798	3631	3571	?	11786
Oocytes collected	1328 (74%)	1849 (66%)	2468 (68%)	2796 (78%)	?	8441 (72%)
Oocytes fertilized	?	?	?	?	?	?
with normal semen						
Oocytes fertilized						
with subnormal semen	?	?	?	?	?	?

Data from QFG unavailable.

Table 5.6. Numbers of patients receiving embryo transfer following oocyte retrieval during standard IVF

	1982	1983	1984	1985	1986	Total
QEH	73	130	202	270	318	993
	103 (71%)	167 (78%)	255 (79%)	307 (88%)	360 (88%)	1192 (83%)
QFG	?	?	523	820	897	2240
			593 (88%)	969 (85%)	1032 (87%)	2594 (86%)
Monash	250	439	529	616	703	2537
	340 (74%)	518 (85%)	607 (87%)	734 (84%)	845 (83%)	3044 (83%)
RNS	101	233	409	469	448	1660
	173 (58%)	296 (79%)	482 (85%)	572 (82%)	526 (85%)	2049 (81%)
RWH	259	324	382	419	?	1384
	336 (77%)	401 (81%)	489 (78%)	491 (85%)		1717 (81%)

Table 5.7. Total pregnancies (including deliveries, abortions, ectoptics and preclinical losses – see Table 5.8 for details) for patients receiving embryo transfer following standard IVF

	1982	1983	1984	1985	1986	Total
QEH	12	29	34	48	74	197
	73 (15%)	130 (22%)	202 (17%)	270 (18%)	318 (23%)	993 (20%)
QFG	?	13	81	138	143	362
		?	523 (15%)	820 (17%)	897 (16%)	2240 (16%)
Monash	45	74	96	113	116	444
	250 (18%)	439 (17%)	529 (18%)	616 (18%)	703 (17%)	2537 (18%)
RNS	7	34	35	54	80	210
	101 (7%)	233 (15%)	409 (9%)	469 (12%)	448 (18%)	1660 (13%)
RWH	55	68	67	106	?	296
	259 (21%)	324 (21%)	382 (18%)	419 (25%)		1384 (21%)

than 2500 g). The perinatal death rate was 47.5 per 1000 births, which is approximately twice that predicted once adjustments for maternal age and multiple pregnancy have been taken into account.

There have been two studies published in the literature dealing with cumulative or life table prospects of pregnancy following multiple attempts at IVF (Kovacs et al. 1986; Guzick et al. 1986). In the first of these studies Kovacs and colleagues found that the cumulative pregnancy rate was 12.9%, 24.6%, 34.7%, 41.2% and 48.6% over the first five cycles respectively. In other words, out of a cohort of 100 women all prepared to undertake five cycles of IVF (unless they became pregnant before five cycles were completed), 48.6% would become pregnant. Similar calculations by Guzick and colleagues gave figures of 13.6%, 24.8%, 37.2%, 47.8% and 52.2%, which are surprisingly similar to those of the Kovacs team. These figures demonstrate that discussions of IVF pregnancy rates should take into account the number of treatment cycles each couple undergo, as well as the success rate on any individual cycle.

Table 5.8 Pregnancy outcome for pregnancies resulting from standard IVF

	1982	1983	1984	1985	1986	Total
QEH						
Delivered	11	19	23	31	57	141 (72%)
Aborted	1	9	20	17	10	47 (24%)
Preclinical	—	—	—	—	4	4 (2%)
Ectopic	0	1	1	0	3	5 (2%)
QFG						
Delivered	—	11	58	94	117	280 (75%)
Aborted	—	2	21	38	25	86 (23%)
Preclinical	—	—	—	—	—	—
Ectopic	—	0	2	6	1	9 (2%)
Monash						
Delivered	28	54	58	67	76	283 (64%)
Aborted	15	15	24	32	29	115 (26%)
Preclinical	0	3	9	5	5	22 (5%)
Ectopic	2	2	5	6	6	22 (5%)
RNS						
Delivered	5	23	25	36	49	138 (66%)
Aborted	1	5	8	17	16	47 (22%)
Preclinical	1	2	1	0	11	15 (7%)
Ectopic	0	4	1	1	4	10 (5%)
RWH						
Delivered	30	35	37	63	?	165 (56%)
Aborted	5	15	11	8	?	39 (13%)
Preclinical	14	13	16	22	?	76 (26%)
Ectopic	6	5	3	2	?	16 (5%)

5.2.4 Gamete Intra-fallopian Transfer

Gamete intra-fallopian transfer (GIFT) became a significant treatment alternative for patients with idiopathic infertility during 1986. Pregnancy rates following GIFT are higher than those for IVF, ranging from 18% to 36% (Table 5.9). It would appear from these results that GIFT should become the first option for

Table 5.9. Results for GIFT treatment cycles during 1986

	QEH	QFG	Monash	RNS	RWH
Patients commencing GIFT treatment	105	95	56	—	237
Oocyte retrievals	86	95	52	147	236
Oocyte replacements	86	95	43[a]	147	236
Pregnancies					
Delivered	25	22	8	19	34
Aborted	3	6	1	4	7
Preclinical	2	—	0	2	7
Ectopic	1	2	0	2	2
Total	31 (36%)	30 (32%)	9 (21%)	27 (18%)	50 (21%)

[a] Nine patients were changed to standard IVF because of signs of tubal abnormality during oocyte retrieval.

those patients for which it is suitable. In addition to the higher success rates, GIFT requires reduced laboratory facilities compared with IVF.

5.2.5 Embryo Cryopreservation

Embryo cryopreservation has not yet proved an effective improvement to the overall success of the IVF procedure (Table 5.10). Most major groups now have embryo freezing facilities and all in this study have reported at least one pregnancy. However, a significant number of embryos (84% to 44%) do not survive the freeze–thaw process, and of those patients that do receive a transfer with frozen embryos the pregnancy rate is in the range of 4%–11%. In extenuation of these apparently low success rates is the practice, observed by most groups, of always transferring the "best" embryos back to the patient during the IVF treatment cycle and only saving those that remain for freezing.

Table 5.10. Embryo cryopreservation statistics

	1982	1983	1984	1985	1986	Totals
QEH						
Patients having embryos frozen	—	7	27	50	69	153
Embryos frozen	—	11	97	158	181	447
Embryos thawed	—	2	86	110	28	226
Embryos surviving thawing	—	0	7	19	10	36 (16%)
Patients having transfer	—	0	4	13	6	23
Pregnancies	—	—	2	1	0	3 (13%)
QFG						
Patients having embryos frozen	—	—	—	40	80	120
Embryos frozen	—	—	—	116	223	339
Embryos thawed	—	—	—	?	175	
Embryos surviving thawing	—	—	—	?	?	
Patients having transfer	—	—	—	6	58	64
Pregnancies	—	—	—	1	6	7 (11%)
Monash						
Patients having embryos frozen	26	96	186	202	140	740
Embryos frozen	40	175	342	453	305	1315
Embryos thawed	23	58	235	251	298	865
Embryos surviving thawing	7	27	123	137	175	469 (54%)
Patients having transfer	7	18	83	90	110	308
Pregnancies	1	8	7	9	1	26 (8%)
RNS						
Patients having embryos frozen	—	—	—	10	87	97
Embryos frozen	—	—	—	17	183	200
Embryos thawed	—	—	—	12	57	69
Embryos surviving thawing	—	—	—	8	31	39 (56%)
Patients having transfer	—	—	—	3	25	28
Pregnancies	—	—	—	0	1	1 (4%)
RWH						
Patients having embryos frozen	—	—	—	—	79	79
Embryos frozen	—	—	—	—	208	208
Embryos thawed	—	—	—	—	68	68
Embryos surviving thawing	—	—	—	—	47	47 (69%)
Patients having transfer	—	—	—	—	32	32
Pregnancies	—	—	—	—	3	3 (9%)

From a moral viewpoint cryopreservation provides an acceptable solution to the problem of dealing with excess embryos that may be produced as a result of the ovulation induction process. This is particularly relevant in view of the increased perinatal mortality that is associated with multiple pregnancies in IVF.

Acknowledgements

The compilation of this chapter would not have been possible without the ready contribution of data from other IVF units. In particular, thanks are due to Dr. Lou Warnes at the Queen Elizabeth Hospital in Adelaide, to Keith Harrison of the Queensland Fertility Group in Brisbane, Dr. Ian Pike at the Royal North Shore Hospital in Sydney and Dr. Ian Johnstone at the Royal Women's Hospital in Melbourne.

References

Cummins JM, Breen TM, Harrison KL et al. (1986) A formula for scoring human embryo growth rates in in vitro fertilization: its value in predicting pregnancy and in comparison with visual estimates of embryo quality. J In Vitro Fert Embryo Transfer 3:284–295

Edmonds DK, Lindsay KS, Miller JF et al. (1982) Early embryonic mortality in women. Fertil Steril 38:447–453

French FE, Bierman JM (1962) Probabilities of fetal mortality. Public Health Rep 77:835

Guzick DS, Wilkes C, Jones HW (1986) Cumulative pregnancy rates for in vitro fertilization. Fertil Steril 46:663–667

Healy DL, Okamoto S, Morrow L et al. (1987) Contributions of in vitro fertilization to knowledge of the reproductive endocrinology of the menstrual cycle. In: Baillière's clinical endocrinology and metabolism, vol 1, no. 1. Baillière, London, pp 133–152

Jones HW Jr, Acosta AA, Andrews MC et al. (1983): What is a pregnancy? : a question for programs of in vitro fertilization. Fertil Steril 40:728–733

Kovacs GT, Rogers P, Leeton JF et al. (1986) In vitro fertilization and embryo transfer. Prospects of pregnancy by life table analysis. Med J Aust 144:682–683

Lenton EA, Osborn J, Fothergill D, Cooke ID (1987) Early pregnancy loss in normal women and following IVF. Presented at the 5th world congress on in vitro fertilization and embryo transfer. Norfolk, Virginia, April 1987

Liu H-C, Rosenwaks Z, Jones HW Jnr (1987) Evidence of early implantation in some IVF non-pregnant patients. Presented at the 5th world congress on in vitro fertilization and embryo transfer. Norfolk, Virginia, April 1987

Martinez F, Trounson AO (1986) An analysis of factors associated with ectopic pregnancy in a human in vitro fertilization programme. Fertil Steril 45:79–87

National Perinatal Statistics Unit (1987) In vitro fertilization pregnancies, Australia and New Zealand 1979–1985. Sydney (ISSN 0816–6889)

Rogers PAW, Milne B, Trounson AO (1986) A model to show uterine receptivity and embryo viability following ovarian stimulation for in vitro fertilization. J In Vitro Fert Embryo Transfer 3:93–98

Veeck LL (1984) Extracorporeal maturation. Ann NY Acad Sci 442:357

Yates CA, De Kretser DM (1987) Male factor infertility and in vitro fertilization. J In Vitro Fert Embryo Transfer 4:141–147

6 Gamete Intra-fallopian Transfer

R. P. S. Jansen

6.1 History

The principle is simple: increase the chance of conception by increasing the concentration of spermatozoa and ova in the fallopian tubes. Direct transfer of gametes to the fallopian tubes was tried in rabbits in the late 1940s (Chang 1982) and in humans by several groups through the 1970s – the years of despair for the scientists and clinicians who were hoping to achieve a human pregnancy by in vitro fertilization (IVF). Occasional pregnancies were then reported in isolated circumstances in which gametes were transferred to the tubes or to the uterus (e.g. Shettles 1979; Craft et al. 1982). However, until the techniques of preparing oocytes and spermatozoa had been refined to the point at which IVF had become clinically successful, it was not realized how carefully gametes must be handled. Oocyte and sperm preparation is as critical for gamete intra-fallopian transfer as it is for IVF.

Once the question of direct tubal transfer of gametes was readdressed in the 1980s by researchers with IVF experience, pregnancies began to follow. The first report that indicated consistent success was published by Asch (Asch et al. 1984). The construction "gamete intra-fallopian transfer" was suggested to Asch by his eldest daughter; thus came about the acronym GIFT. GIFT is now widely accepted as denoting the two-step procedure of follicle aspiration for oocyte collection and then transfer of oocytes and capacitated spermatozoa deep into the ampulla of the tube, close to the ampullary–isthmic junction, utilizing laparoscopy (Asch et al. 1985, 1986a; Nemiro and McGaughey 1986; Molloy et al. 1986; Guastella et al. 1986; Corson et al. 1986), mini-laparotomy (Asch et al. 1986b), or recently ultrasound (Jansen and Anderson 1987) to catheterize the tube.

6.2 Gamete Preparation

6.2.1 Ovarian Stimulation and Laparoscopic Follicle Aspiration

GIFT, like IVF, demands multiple oocytes for clinical efficacy. Intentional ovarian hyperstimulation with clomiphene and pituitary gonadotrophins

Table 6.1. Sperm penetration of immature and mature human oocytes

Oocyte stage	% sperm entry	Subsequent cleavage
Primary oocyte		
Germinal vesicle	16.7	No
Germinal vesicle breakdown	25.0	No
Metaphase I	34.8	No
Secondary oocyte		
Metaphase II	66.7	Yes

From Lopata 1985.

(Chap. 2) is the same for GIFT as it is for IVF. But GIFT differs from IVF in that eggs, to be useful, probably need to be immediately preovulatory, secondary oocytes at the time of follicle aspiration and transfer to the tubes, whereas less mature eggs for fertilization in the laboratory can be developed further in vitro before sperm are introduced. Premature penetration of eggs by spermatozoa, before the eggs reach metaphase of the second meiotic division, prevents subsequent development. Table 6.1 summarizes Lopata's data on the ability of spermatozoa to penetrate immature eggs in vitro: the data should apply equally to fertilization in vivo and emphasize the need for eggs transferred to the tubes with capacitated spermatozoa to be as mature as possible. At Sydney IVF we therefore carry out laparoscopy for follicle aspiration 38 hours from the time of administration of human chorionic gonadotrophin (hCG). The procedure of securing oocytes for GIFT is otherwise the same as it is for IVF (Chap. 3).

As laparoscopy is giving way in IVF programmes to ultrasound-based follicle aspiration, so interest is waning in studying the effects of the physical and chemical environment to which laparoscopically collected oocytes are exposed. Ultrasound-guided transvaginal follicle aspiration in conscious patients avoids untoward actions of systemic anaesthetic drugs (except those of local anaesthetic agents), pelvic cooling from the pneumoperitoneum, metabolic acidosis of the pelvic environment from absorption of carbon dioxide (CO_2), and trauma to the ovarian ligaments from intraoperative manipulation. The new popularity of laparoscopy-based GIFT procedures, however, emphasizes the lasting importance of these variables. Because GIFT can technically be carried out without the training and equipment so obviously necessary for IVF, the physical and chemical hazards to oocytes that attend laparoscopy should be appreciated and studied further.

Preovulatory maturation of the follicle follows the mid-cycle gonadotrophin peak or the administration of human chorionic gonadotrophin (hCG) (Chap. 2). The oocyte's first meiotic division is completed as part of this process of maturation and the second meiotic division starts. In preparation for ovulation, the follicular cells of the cumulus oophorus produce highly acidic glycosaminoglycans, including chondroitin sulphate (Eppig 1979; Ax and Ryan 1979), which occupy huge domains of water, causing the fluid between the cumulus cells to undergo a change from a solution to a mucus-like gel and causing the space between the follicular cells to expand (Eppig 1980). The expanded cumulus mass at or near ovulation is a macroscopic structure a millimetre or more in diameter. The cumulus can be expected to be an important chemical and physical buffer for the oocyte in its contact with the abnormal environment of a GIFT procedure.

The oocyte's environment is disturbed when laparoscopy begins. General anaesthesia involves administration of, typically, the following sequence of drugs:

1. A short-acting barbiturate such as thiopentone for induction of anaesthesia.
2. A muscle relaxant, either a competitive blocking agent in the case of *d*-tubocurarine, atracurium or alcuronium, or a depolarizing (and potassium-releasing) agent such as suxamethonium.
3. Nitrous oxide mixed with oxygen.
4. A volatile inhalational agent such as halothane or enflurane.
5. Neostigmine and atropine to reverse the effects of non-depolarizing muscle relaxants.
6. Supplemental narcotic or non-narcotic analgesics, administered before, during and after the procedure.

A local anaesthetic drug such as xylocaine or bupivicaine may be used as an adjunct for laparoscopy or may be the main anaesthetic agent for ultrasound-based follicle aspiration. Unlike IVF, in which oocytes are isolated quickly and perhaps can be freed from the effects of these drugs, GIFT involves a return of gametes to the reproductive tract while the effects of the drugs are still apparent. Data on the effects of these drugs on oocyte and sperm function are scanty and mostly indirect.

Wikland (1987) found that follicular fluid xylocaine concentrations after infiltration of the vagina with 5 ml 1% xylocaine approximated 0.4 μg/ml. In producing local anaesthesia, xylocaine's pharmacological action involves its stabilization of cell membranes, preventing nerve depolarization. Depolarizing events that are important to reproduction include the acrosome reaction and fertilization itself. Sperm movement is so slowed by local anaesthetic drugs in high concentration that inhibition of sperm motility has been proposed as a general bioassay for their membrane stabilizing activity (Hong et al. 1981). The concentration of xylocaine that decreases sperm motility to 50% of that in control samples, however, is 18 mmol/l (Hong et al. 1986), or 1.87 mg/ml. Whereas IVF procedures are little influenced by transient oocyte contact with xylocaine, the same may not necessarily be true when oocytes and sperm are placed immediately in the well-vascularized fallopian tubes, where locally absorbed drug could be active at the time of, for example, GIFT procedures carried out ultrasonographically.

Intravenously administered barbiturates also enter ovarian follicles before aspiration can be carried out; follicular fluid concentrations increase steadily during the course of laparoscopy (Endler et al. 1987). We have found, however, no evidence to show that the duration of GIFT laparoscopies adversely affects clinical pregnancy rates (Fig. 6.1). Fertilizability of oocytes has been claimed to be lower for follicles aspirated towards the end of laparoscopic egg pickup procedures when compared with those aspirated at once (Hayes et al. 1987; Go et al. 1987), but reported differences are trivial and may be accounted for by the operator's tendency to aspirate smaller, less obvious, and probably less optimal follicles last. These same data can also be interpreted to suggest that nitrous oxide, too, has no cumulatively deleterious effect on oocyte function during GIFT; repeated exposure of male mice to 50% nitrous oxide over 14 weeks has no apparently harmful effect on sperm production (Mazze et al. 1983).

The volatile inhalational drugs halothane, enflurane and methoxyflurane cause

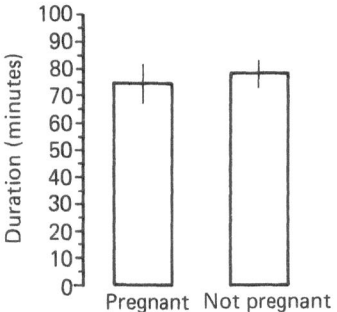

Fig. 6.1. Duration of GIFT laparoscopies (median and 95% confidence limits of median) in pregnancy cycles and non-pregnancy cycles at Sydney IVF ($n=150$).

rapid induction of the acrosome reaction in sea urchin spermatozoa (Hinkley et al. 1986). The effect, interestingly, is blocked by the local anaesthetic drug procaine. Halothane has been shown also to inhibit sperm–egg binding and to predispose to polyspermic fertilization and abnormal cleavage of sea urchin eggs (Hinkley et al. 1986; Hinkley and Wright 1986). It is prudent to minimize the use of these inhalational agents in GIFT laparoscopies, especially towards the end of the procedure when the gametes are due to be transferred. Pregnancy rates in our series at Sydney IVF were higher if a supplementary parenteral agent such as fentanyl, droperidol or pethidine had been administered prior to or during laparoscopy, meaning perhaps that these patients were exposed to lower concentrations of inhalational anaesthetic drugs.

I have found no data to relate muscle relaxant drugs to effects on reproductive function. At Sydney IVF, pregnancies have occurred despite our occasional need to use suxamethonium at the time of gamete transfer to the tubes. Potassium levels rise when muscle depolarization takes place after administration of suxamethonium. The fallopian tube lumen normally has a potassium concentration of 20 mequiv/l or higher (Borland et al. 1980), so a hyperkalaemic environment will probably do no harm at the time of transfer.

The oocyte is known to exhibit acetylcholine receptors of muscarinic type, which would be expected to be blocked by atropine. Initial depolarization of the oocyte with sperm–egg fusion has been attributed to activation of these receptors. There was no dose–effect relationship evident between neostigmine, atropine and pregnancy rates in a small number of patients studied at Sydney IVF, but because neostigmine and atropine are given at the end of a GIFT procedure – just when sperm–egg interactions are commencing – systematic studies on the effects of muscle relaxants and atropine on fertilization in vitro and in vivo may be rewarding.

The cumulus oophorus is an important physical and chemical buffer for the oocyte. The relative robustness of GIFT procedures compared with IVF, and GIFT's higher pregnancy rate, may in part be attributable to the oocyte's additional layer of protection during pickup, examination and transfer in comparison with embryos, which are protected only by the zona pellucida during the time of transfer from laboratory to uterus.

Although it is often thought that vacuum pressures need to be monitored carefully during follicle aspiration, there is evidence that the oocyte can withstand considerable accelerative forces yet retain ability to develop normally after fertilization. In a study in which fertilized mouse oocytes at the pronuclear stage were centrifuged at accelerative forces of 25 000 g for 10 minutes (Nakamura et al. 1986), there was redistribution of some cytoplasmic components (pronuclei were visibly more distinct than in uncentrifuged eggs), but further development was possible and normal offspring resulted. It is unlikely that an oocyte cushioned by cumulus would be subjected to these g-forces during ordinary follicle aspiration. Tesarik and colleagues (Tesarik et al. 1980) found no ultrastructural abnormalities in human oocytes obtained at pressures ranging from 7 to 20 mmHg (95–270 mmH$_2$O). Needle effects such as stripping of the cumulus oophorus and fracture of the zona need to be avoided and may be more common with finer needles, with syringe suction, or with follicle flushing (Cohen et al. 1986), but these are consequences that, if they happen, are obvious immediately.

Loss of heat can be harmful for oocytes during meiosis (Karp and Smith 1975). Cooling over 3 hours to an average nadir of 26.4 °C, followed by warming over 2 hours, produced chromosomal abnormalities in 28%–54% of sheep oocytes cooled at all stages of meiosis from germinal vesicle breakdown to metaphase II (Moor and Crosby 1985). Abnormalities included disorganization of metaphase plates and the development of multipolar spindles. These abnormalities take place because low-temperature-induced disassembly of microtubules through depolymerization of the major structural protein of microtubules, tubulin (Petzelt 1979), is then followed by faulty repolymerization and microtubule redevelopment as the temperature rises again. Few data are available on the short but sharp cooling that might accompany follicle aspiration with the low environmental temperatures likely to be encountered during follicle aspiration for GIFT. The cumulus oophorus would have little effect in insulating the oocyte against cooling, so it is prudent to take exceptional precautions to maintain the temperature of oocytes during collection, examination and transfer.

Laparoscopy means insufflation of the peritoneum with gas, usually 100% CO_2, which forms carbonic acid in solution. Oocytes, or more correctly the oocyte–cumulus complexes, are exposed to substantial pH changes during oocyte pickup. Movement in pH away from the physiological range (pH 7.4 to 7.5) has harmful effects on fertilization rates in vitro and on subsequent cleavage. For example, mouse oocytes in culture medium acidified to pH 6.9 by contact with 20% CO_2 for 1 hour show morphological evidence of cytolysis, a higher proportion of polypronuclear fertilization than controls, and a lower chance of reaching the 2-cell stage; alkaline pH extremes (pH 7.8) induce cleavage arrest at a later stage of cleavage, with inhibition of blastocyst formation (Puissant et al. 1986).

Because the duration of laparoscopy with 100% CO_2 for pneumoperitoneum has no major influence on oocyte fertilization rates (Fig. 6.1), it is unlikely that significant pH changes take place in follicular fluid prior to aspiration. Although some absorption of CO_2 occurs from the peritoneal cavity into the circulation, the effects of this absorption on blood are negligible and easily overcome by moderate hyperventilation (Seed et al. 1970). The point at which contact of eggs with CO_2 occurs is when the oocyte–cumulus complex enters the collection needle and tubing; at this time the needle is often withdrawn from the follicle and peritoneal gas is used to complete the aspiration. Aspiration of CO_2 is inevitable also when the operator observes the mucus of a cumulus complex at the aspiration site or on the surface of an ovulating follicle. Follicular fluid, CO_2-bicarbonate-based buffers and phosphate-based buffers all show falls in pH to below the physiological range within 2 minutes of exposure to 100% CO_2 (Chetkowski et al. 1985); in one clinical series, follicular fluid aspirated in ordinary circumstances showed pH values in the range 6.87 to 7.42, with a mean of 7.16 (Bize et al. 1987); we have found the same at Sydney IVF (Fig. 6.2).

How can the oocyte be protected from the effects of CO_2? It is likely that the highly expanded cumulus matrix, which consists of sulphated glycosaminogly-cans, and the zona pellucida, which is composed of slightly less acidic, sialyated mucus glycoproteins, effectively retard acidification of the oocyte itself. In other words, the oocyte in cumulus is shielded from the effects of a falling pH either of the follicular fluid or of the medium into which the cumulus–oocyte complex is collected, provided that exposure to CO_2 is shortlived. Unfortunately, simply replacing aspirated CO_2 in the collection tube with aspirated room air before sealing the tube and sending it for examination has little effect on the pH of received follicular fluid.

Alternatively, 5% CO_2 (the same gas used in IVF incubators) can be used for pneumoperitoneum (Edwards and Steptoe 1983; Urry et al. 1987). This substitution effectively prevents the acidification of aspirated fluid and of peritoneal fluid (Fig. 6.2). But how harmful is transient acidification of the fluid environment of the oocyte–cumulus complex? In one study in which 100% CO_2 was used for pneumoperitoneum, oocytes recovered at laparoscopy from CO_2-affected perito-neal fluid (fluid that from our studies would have an expected pH significantly less than follicular fluid – Fig. 6.2) were as likely to be fertilized as were oocytes recovered from intact follicles (Matson et al. 1986). Although a residue of acidic peritoneal fluid after gamete transfer to the tubes for GIFT, as opposed to IVF, could possibly harm the intratubal environment at the time of fertilization, no studies exist on intratubal pH changes during and after GIFT with 100% CO_2 for the pneumoperitoneum; but at Sydney IVF the pregnancy rate with GIFT has been no different with 100% or 5% CO_2. It has long been known that the efficient respiratory removal of CO_2 by assisted ventilation is effective during laparoscopy in preventing acidosis of arterial blood (Seed et al. 1970) and, presumably, of well-vascularised tissues such as the fallopian tubes.

The main disadvantages of using air or predominantly air for pneumoperito-neum instead of 100% CO_2 result from nitrogen's slow absorption into solution in comparison with absorption of CO_2. With air there is a higher incidence of postoperative shoulder pain caused by retained gas under the diaphragm. In the rare event that gas embolism should occur, there is a greater likelihood with nitrogen that the clinical situation would be irretrievable and that death rather than recovery would follow.

Until controlled studies are done to compare the effects of air versus CO_2 on the intratubal environment or pregnancy rates with GIFT, no confident recom-mendation can be made on which gas should be used for the pneumoperitoneum.

Changes in pH during examination of follicular fluid and during isolation of oocytes before transfer depend on the nature of the buffering medium used and the gas in contact with it. Bicarbonate ion is necessary for oocytes to be fertilized (Lee and Storey 1986). This need lies behind the choice of 5% CO_2-bicarbonate buffers such as Ham's F10 and Whittingham's T6 for IVF-related work, and this experience in turn has led to the use of CO_2-bicarbonate buffer systems for GIFT. In air, these buffers show pH rises to alkaline levels (Bourne 1986), so a 5% CO_2

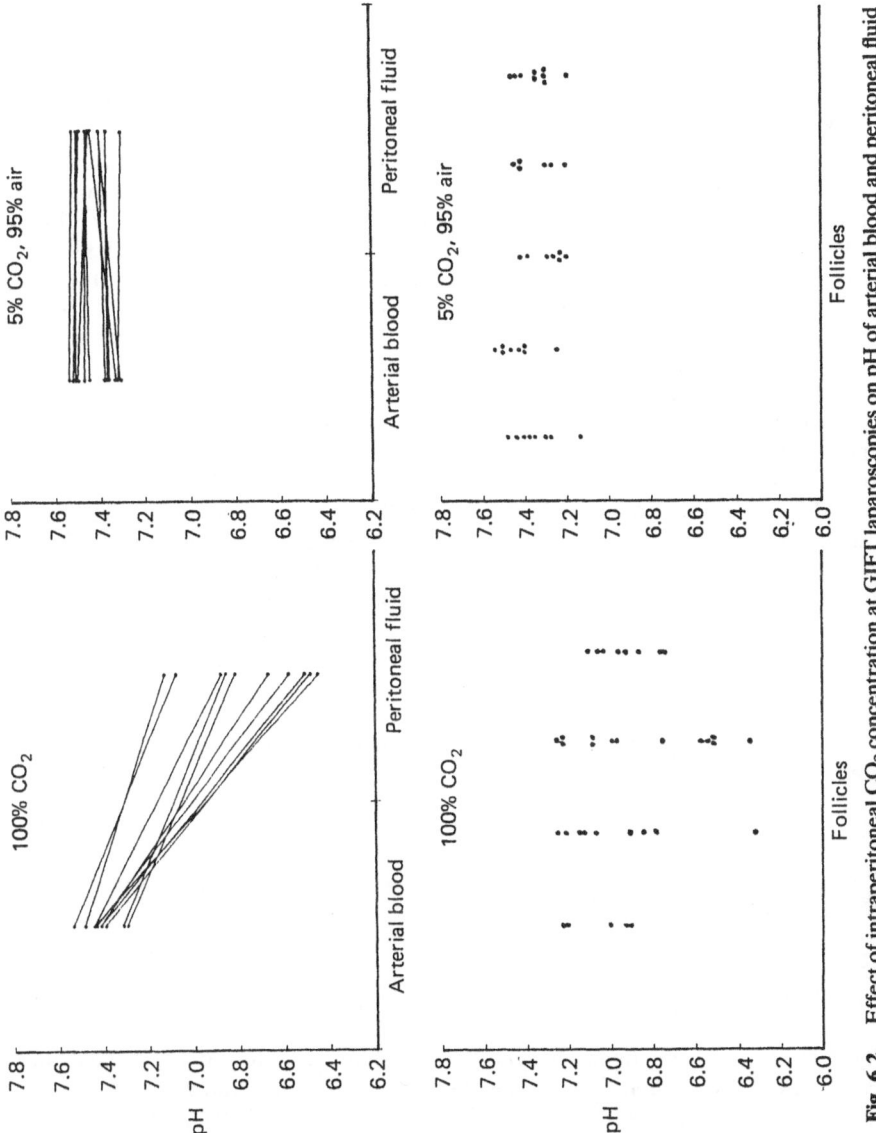

Fig. 6.2. Effect of intraperitoneal CO_2 concentration at GIFT laparoscopies on pH of arterial blood and peritoneal fluid (paired samples, *above*) and on pH of aspirated fluid from multiple follicles (individual cases, *below*).

environment is usually devised for examining follicular fluid for oocytes and for holding oocytes in buffer prior to transfer.

6.2.2 Preparation of Spermatozoa

The aim of sperm preparation for GIFT is to cause capacitation of spermatozoa without inducing acrosome reactions. Once capacitated, sperm show accelerated motility and acquire the ability to attach to the zona pellucida, at which point the acrosome reaction should occur for penetration of the zona pellucida (Overstreet et al. 1987). No systematic studies have examined the effectiveness of current sperm centrifugation and swim-up procedures in achieving these aims. Instead, the procedures known to be effective for sperm capacitation prior to IVF have been used for GIFT. Sperm capacitation for intratubal fertilization may involve different principles to the requirements for IVF. Although there is no firm empirical basis for the suggestion that spermatozoa should be prepared 2.5 hours prior to a GIFT laparoscopy (Asch 1987), the discovery, almost 40 years ago, of the need mammalian spermatozoa have for capacitation prior to attainment of fertilizing capacity came from the observation that the transfer of fresh sperm and eggs to rabbit tubes was not followed by conception (Chang 1982).

The number of motile spermatozoa transferred to the fallopian tubes at GIFT is about 100 000 per tube (Asch et al. 1985; Yovich et al. 1986), in a volume of 25–30 μl. At fertilization after sexual intercourse the spermatozoa in the ampulla of the tube number fewer than 100 (Chang 1982) and the volume of intratubular fluid is negligible. Despite its clinical usefulness, GIFT falls short of mimicking natural circumstances in the tubes. Yovich has found that even when 100 000 motile sperm can be transferred for couples in whom the male partner has oligospermia the pregnancy rate is still lower than when men with normal semen analyses are involved (Yovich et al. 1986). Better results may follow when several-fold higher numbers of sperm are transferred (Blackledge et al. 1986), the role of GIFT in overcoming infertility due partly or wholly to male factors is limited.

6.3   Gamete Transfer

6.3.1 Laparoscopy

Several catheters have been designed to transfer gametes to the tubes once oocytes have been identified and isolated and the spermatozoa have been prepared. They are generally about 16-French in gauge and 60 cm in length (e.g. Intracath, Deseret; GIFT catheter, William Cook).

Asch described the technique of loading the catheter as follows (Asch et al. 1984). The catheter, fitted with a 1 ml tuberculin syringe (or a finer syringe such as a Hamilton syringe) at one end, is rinsed twice with Ham's F10 or similar medium and loaded in this sequence: 10 μl Ham's F10, an air space of 5 μl, 25 μl of the sperm preparation containing 100 000 sperm, another air space of 5 μl, two oocytes loaded in 40 μl medium, another air space of 5 μl, and finally another 10 μl medium. Molloy et al. (1986) used a similar loading procedure. At Sydney IVF we now load the catheters without air, and with smaller volumes of medium, depending on the sperm concentration (aiming still to transfer 100 000 sperm per tube); gametes for both tubes are loaded sequentially into the one catheter and a Hamilton syringe is used for accurate transfer of required volumes.

Catheterization of the tubes at laparoscopy is difficult. Palmer forceps or similar instruments are used to secure the fallopian tube, either by pinching a small amount of serosa close to the fimbrial end or by encompassing the tube at the infundibulum. Air left at the end of the transfer catheter is expelled on the fimbrial surface. The catheter is then manipulated into the ampulla. If the infundibulum has been surrounded by the grasping forceps the catheter travels between the jaws of the forceps. The catheter is passed a distance of 2–6 cm, essentially to the ampullary–isthmic junction, although convolutions of the tube may not always allow this without risking trauma to the mucosa.

It cannot be stressed too greatly that the gametes must not be expelled until the operator is sure that the catheter is deep inside the lumen of the tube; extraluminal placement, through the fimbriae, and despite tubal movement on moving the catheter, is a simple reason for GIFT to fail. There should be no hurry to transfer the gametes: we have found no association between the time taken to transfer and the pregnancy rate. A quadruplet pregnancy has occurred at Sydney IVF after a transfer that, before the first tube was successfully catheterized, involved the lapse of 20 minutes and the relocation of the abdominal site for the transfer catheter before the four oocytes reached the tube.

6.3.2 Minilaparotomy

Some of the early pregnancies that followed GIFT were obtained not through laparoscopy but by way of suprapubic minilaparotomy (Asch et al. 1985, 1986b). Once the small, horizontal, suprapubic incision has been made and the peritoneal cavity has been entered, instruments similar to those for laparoscopy are used for aspirating follicles and then for cannulating the tubes for gamete transfer. Minilaparotomy avoids the possible gametopathic effects of CO_2-peritoneum. Pregnancy rates are at least as good as with laparoscopy, but patients' acceptance of minilaparotomy as a repeated technique, should pregnancy not occur immediately, is limited. Few GIFT units nowadays use this means of recovering oocytes and transferring gametes.

6.3.3 Transvaginal GIFT

Transvaginal ultrasound-guided follicle aspiration under local anaesthesia for obtaining oocytes for IVF is now well described and widely practised (Chap. 3). Little or no systemic sedation or analgesia is needed, so the possibly harmful effects of general anaesthesia on oocytes can be avoided. Transvaginal oocyte recovery has been followed by IVF and then early, pronuclear-stage, transfer of fertilized eggs to the fallopian tubes at laparoscopy (Blackledge et al. 1986; Devroey, et al. 1986; Yovich et al. 1987; Silber et al. 1987). Speculation has followed on the possibility that gamete transfer or pronuclear-stage egg transfer to the tubes might be able to be accomplished transvaginally.

In 1987 we described a reliable means for catheterizing the fallopian tubes from the vagina, using a transvaginal ultrasound probe to guide a firm outer cannula into the lateral uterine angle, after which a 2-French inner catheter is advanced through the uterotubal junction and into the tubal isthmus (Jansen and Anderson 1987). The procedure is shown in Fig. 6.3. By transferring spermatozoa just before spontaneous ovulation, we increased the pregnancy rate in a donor insemination programme five-fold higher than that we had achieved with timed intracervical inseminations (Jansen et al. 1988a). GIFT too may be able to be carried out by ultrasound using local anaesthesia instead of by laparoscopy using general anaesthesia.

Such non-operative tubal gamete transfer, or "ultrasound-GIFT", would allow greater flexibility in varying the timing of the transfer according to circumstances. Oocyte maturity, for example, can be judged after aspiration; if incomplete, maturity can be reached in vitro before transfer. Furthermore, in cases of oligospermia, or whenever fertilization cannot be taken for granted, oocytes can

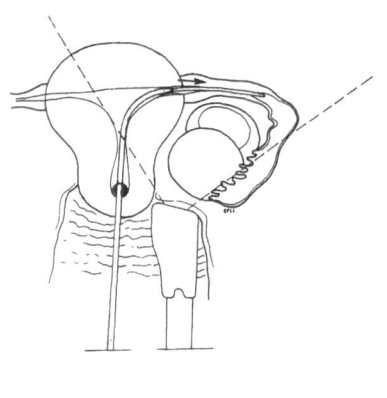
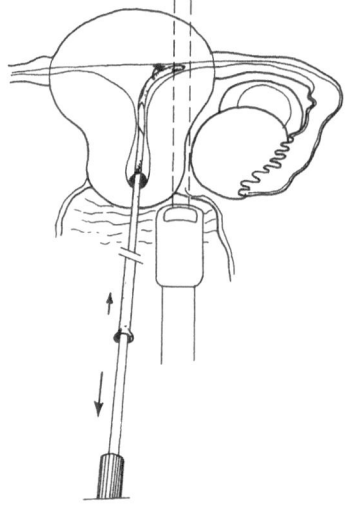

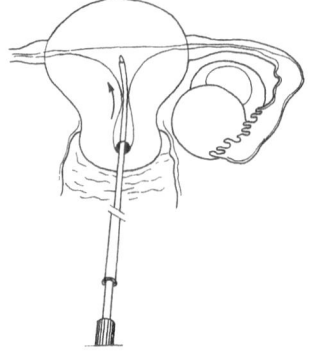

Fig. 6.3. Techniques of catheterization of the fallopian tubes from the vagina, guided by intravaginal ultrasound. **a** (top left) The outer cannula is guided into the uterus, helped if necessary with a metal obturator at right angles to the lateral curve of the cannula. **b** (top right) As the obturator is withdrawn, the cannula regains its lateral curve and is advanced to the uterotubal junction, where it is visualized by ultrasound. **c** (bottom right) The inner catheter is passed down the cannula and through the isthmus of the tube. (From Jansen and Anderson (1987). Reprinted with permission.)

be fertilized in vitro and then transferred 18–20 hours later, when they are at the pronuclear stage – a procedure already popular at laparoscopy (Blackledge et al. 1986; Devroey et al. 1986; Yovich et al. 1987; Silber et al. 1987). Tubal embryo transfer, whether by laparoscopy or by transuterine tubal catheterization, means that some advantage can still be obtained from the normal tube's embryotrophic properties before the embryo or embryos enter the uterus.

The hope for the future for procedures designed to assist conception is that maximum use will be able to be made in individual couples of whatever normal reproductive components are identified. At the time of writing, we have achieved one pregnancy with IVF and pronuclear-stage transfer to the tubes by ultrasound-guided catheterization of the tubes from the vagina (Jansen et al. 1988b). Work is proceeding on exploring the possibility that transvaginal ovum or pronuclear-stage transfer to the tubes might lead to a routine nonsurgical means of carrying out GIFT. The choice between IVF-uterine embryo transfer and tubal transfer of gametes or zygotes can be expected to depend on increasingly sophisticated ways of assessing the endosalpingeal normality of the fallopian tube.

6.4   Results

6.4.1   Pregnancies and Pregnancy Outcomes

Successful pregnancies after GIFT depend on: (a) paying attention to sterilization of instruments, rinsing of catheters, preparation of gametes and the technique of tubal catheterization and transfer, (b) the number of oocytes that are transferred and (c) the age, the length of previous infertility, and the diagnosis of the woman being treated. Many of these factors also govern the relative incidence of spontaneous abortion.

Tubal pregnancies complicate about 5.6% of clinically apparent conceptions after GIFT, and may be as high as 30% when there is intrinsic or extrinsic tubal disease short of complete tubal occlusion (National Perinatal Statistics Unit and Fertility Society of Australia 1987). Multiple pregnancies may occur in which there is more than one ectopic pregnancy or in which an ectopic pregnancy accompanies one or more intra-uterine pregnancies.

GIFT should provide a higher pregnancy rate and a lower spontaneous abortion rate than IVF does, both within an IVF–GIFT unit and when comparisons are made between programmes (Jansen 1988). The basis for the better pregnancy outcome with GIFT rests on two considerations. Firstly, when normal fallopian tubes are made use of in the reproductive process, physiological circumstances for fertilization and early development of the zygote are likely to be better than when laboratory incubators substitute for the tubes. Secondly, oocytes in cumulus are better protected from adverse environmental conditions during transfer to the tubes than embryos in vitro, protected only by their zona pellucida, are during transfer to the uterus.

Empirically, the collected incidence of clinical and subclinical abortions among uterine pregnancies in GIFT programmes in Australia from 1985 to 1986 was 29.8%, compared with an incidence over the same period with IVF of 35.1%

(National Perinatal Statistics Unit and Fertility Society of Australia 1987). The clinical abortion incidence varied with age, and was, excluding subclinical abortions, 18.1% for women under 30 years, 19.6% for women aged 30 to 34 years, and 25.4% for women aged 35 to 39 years. Almost all GIFT pregnancies in women over 40 years have apparently resulted in abortion.

6.4.2 Effect of Technical Factors

The relative incidence of spontaneous abortion among pregnancies achieved after GIFT treatment provides a more accurate and more sensitive index of success for comparison between and within series than simple pregnancy rates do (Jansen 1982, 1988). An increase in spontaneous abortions among pregnancies in relatively young women receiving GIFT is an early sign that a GIFT programme is technically unsound.

Without duplication of the careful preparative techniques needed for IVF, pregnancy rates with GIFT will at best be suboptimal and at worst will approach zero. At Sydney IVF a nadir of pregnancies occurred for several months while instrument preparation methods were inadvertently changed from autoclaving and washing, to autoclaving alone (with precipitation, it was thought, of minerals onto surfaces in contact with gametes), and then to thorough cleansing and rinsing with highly purified water prior to dry-heat sterilization. The combined clinical and subclinical abortion rate during these three periods went from medium (35%) to high (55%) to low (25%).

6.4.3 Effect of Oocyte Number

Doubling the number of oocytes available for fertilization should roughly double the chance of conception and thus double the chance of pregnancy in any one ovarian cycle. Figure 6.4 shows that part of the efficacy of GIFT procedures lies in exploiting this principle.

Because the number of oocytes transferred during GIFT is typically four (two oocytes to each tube), a false sense of complacency in relation to present GIFT techniques may be fostered if a GIFT pregnancy rate of, say, 25% per treatment cycle is regarded as being comparable to a normal pregnancy rate of 25% per month. If account is also taken of the need for 100 000 sperm per tube for successful GIFT when compared with normal mammalian tubal sperm numbers of fewer than 100 at conception (Chang 1982), the disturbed physiology that attends present GIFT procedures is seen in still starker perpective.

Because high oocyte numbers means introducing the hazard of high multiple pregnancy, improving pregnancy rates by means other than increasing gamete numbers is a high priority for research. Meanwhile, however, the choice of how many oocytes to transfer will remain a means for varying the clinical efficacy of GIFT procedures: this number will depend on the other factors governing success in a particular programme and for a particular couple. The present modal number of oocytes transferred is, in an overwhelming number of published series, four.

Among 173 GIFT pregnancies of at least 20 weeks' gestation in Australia conceived during the years 1985 and 1986 (National Perinatal Statistics Unit and Fertility Society of Australia 1987), more than four oocytes were transferred in

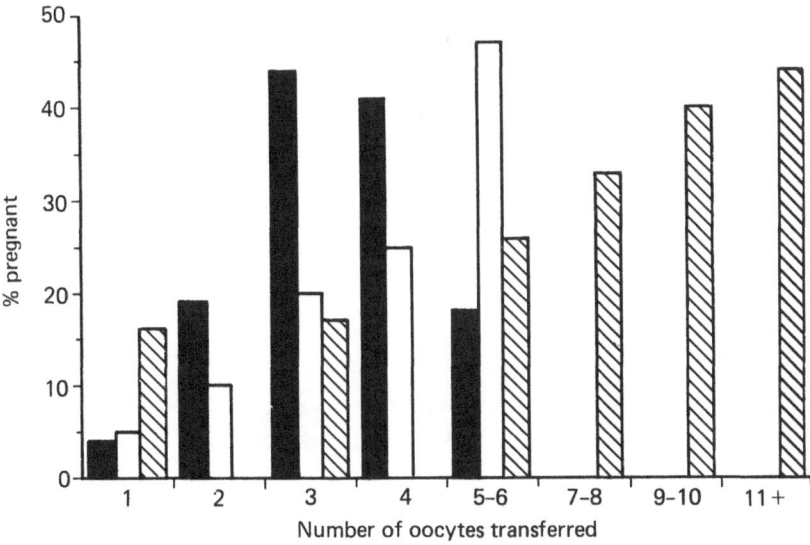

Fig. 6.4. GIFT pregnancy rates per treatment cycle according to number of oocytes transferred in three series: International Cooperative Study (Asch 1987) (*black bars*), Sydney IVF (*white bars*), Humana Hospital Programme (Craft et al. 1987) (*hatched bars*).

only 6.5% of conceptual cycles. Of the 173, 126 (72.8%) were singletons, 39 (22.5%) were twins, and 8 (4.6%) were triplets. Of the 39 twins, 21 (54%) occurred with four oocytes transferred, and 3 (8%) occurred with five or more ocytes transferred. Of the 8 triplets, 2 each occurred with three oocytes transferred, four oocytes transferred and five oocytes transferred, and 1 with more than five oocytes transferred. Limiting the number of oocytes transferred to four would have diminished the birth number of just 3 of the sets of twins and 3 of the sets of triplets. However, it should be remembered that assisted conception procedures such as GIFT already dominate the aetiology of triplets and higher multiples in cities with such infertility programmes, straining those cities' capacity for the medical care of premature neonates.

The argument for increasing oocyte numbers above four when conditions are thought to be adverse for conception (Craft et al. 1987) will need to be balanced not just by the empirically quantifiable risk of multiple pregnancy: the qualitative hazard of high multiple pregnancy, in which none may reach viability, must also be taken into account. In older women, one should consider, too, the special dilemma presented by a twin pregnancy in which one fetus is chromosomally normal on prenatal diagnostic karyotyping and the other is abnormal.

6.4.4   Effect of Clinical Variables

GIFT pregnancy rates vary inversely with the duration of infertility (Fig. 6.5) and also with the age of the patient. Pregnancy rates are in general lower for women with primary infertility than for women with secondary infertility, but much of the effect of previous fertility is lost if the duration of infertility is accounted for.

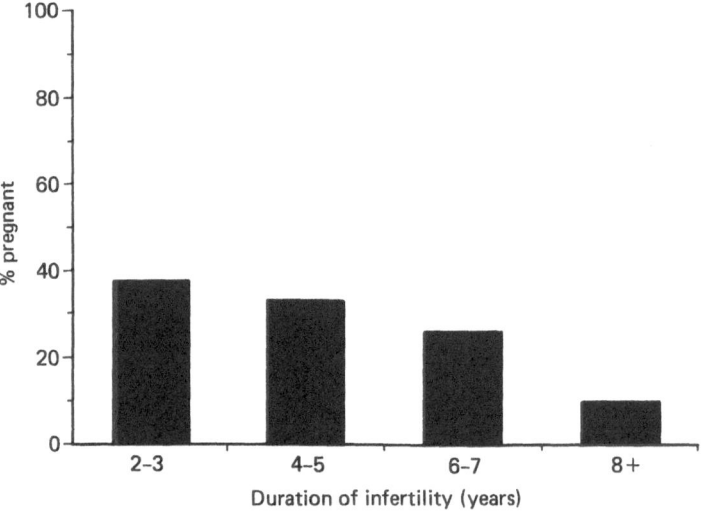

Fig. 6.5. GIFT pregnancy per treatment cycle according to duration of infertility, among patients aged 38 years or less, at Sydney IVF ($n=100$).

Figure 6.6 shows the effect of the cause of infertility on pregnancy rates in two series. Highest pregnancy rates may occur with clear cases of cervical factor or when a normal tube is adherent to the ovarian surface after an ovarian operation. These are situations where intratubal reproductive function is potentially normal and the cause of the infertility is purely one of sperm transport or oocyte pickup; both these situations, however, are relatively uncommon. Average pregnancy rates accompany unexplained infertility and partially-treated, or relatively mild, endometriosis. Untreated severe endometriosis, however, has a negative effect on pregnancy rates and may increase the chance of spontaneous abortion.

Lower than average pregnancy rates accompany oligospermia and intrinsic fallopian tube disease. The observation that poor sperm motility is not readily overcome by GIFT is disappointing, given the prevalence of oligospermia and the intuitive appeal direct tubal transfer of oocytes and spermatozoa has for this condition. Because of the high incidence of tubal pregnancy when GIFT has been used to treat mild fallopian tube disease, a past history of ectopic pregnancy, even if the remaining tube appears normal at laparoscopy and on hysterosalpingography, should usually mean IVF rather than GIFT.

6.5 Complications

The complications of GIFT include the complications of ovarian stimulation (Chap. 2), the complications of operation and laparoscopic or transvaginal follicle aspiration (Chap. 3), and the psychological effects of disappointment (Chap. 12).

The incidence of spontaneous abortion is lower for GIFT (30%) than it is for IVF (35%), but it is considerably higher than it is for normal women (10%–15%), for women receiving intracervical insemination (10%–15%), and for women being treated with menopausal gonadotrophins for anovulation (about 20%) (Jansen 1982). The causes of this increased incidence of abortion may be attributable to a combination of the effects of hyperstimulation on oocyte selection and on tubal and endometrial function, mismatching of oocyte and sperm maturation, polyspermic fertilization, physical injury to oocytes caused by

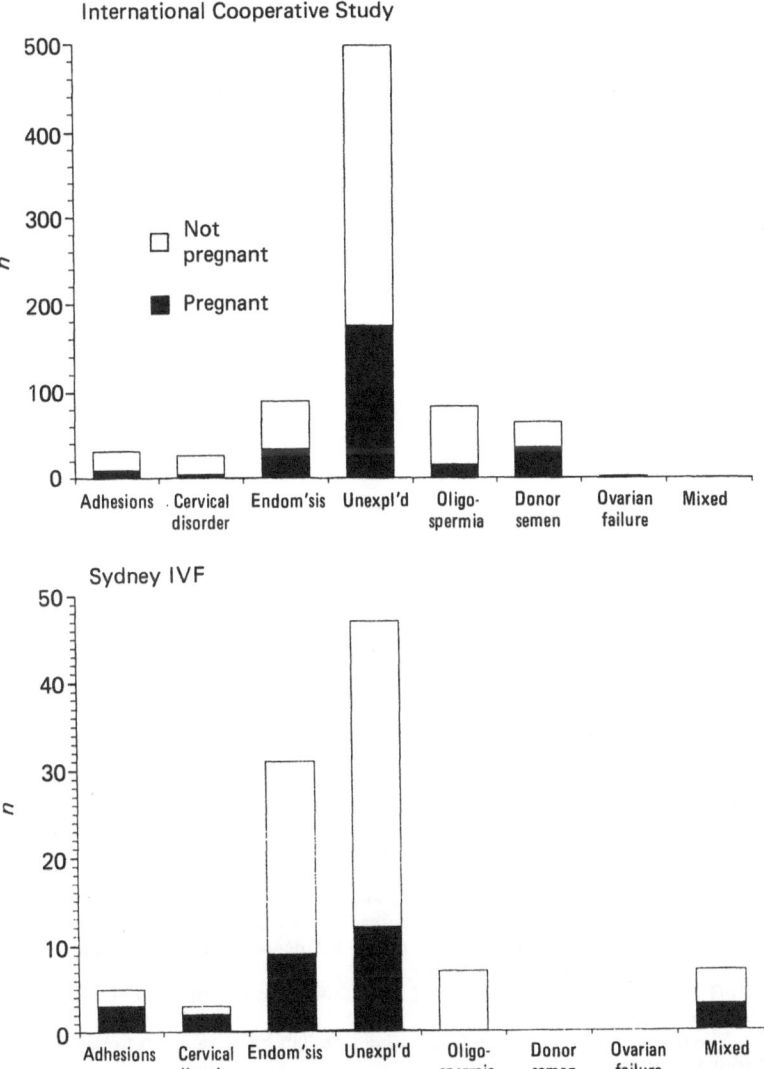

Fig. 6.6. GIFT pregnancies per treatment cycle according to the cause of infertility in two series: an International Cooperative Study coordinated by Asch (1987) ($n=800$), and the first 100 cases of Sydney IVF.

cooling and warming, shifts in pH and exposure to light, and chemical injury to oocytes or the subsequent embryo by shortcomings in the transfer medium, especially contamination of instruments or catheters with nonpurified water.

Multiple pregnancy is a feature that all successful GIFT programmes have in common. Consideration should be given to transferring fewer oocytes when infertility is of relatively short duration or when a patient is only in her twenties, as the chance of successful conception is high in such patients.

Ectopic pregnancy is predisposed to by the effect of hyperstimulation (McBain et al. 1980) and, especially, by the presence of intrinsic tubal disease. The effect of extrinsic tubal disease, namely peritubal adhesions or adherences between tube and ovary, is less certain in the absence of endosalpingeal damage. The question of the presence or absence of minimal tubal disease will become especially important as the procedure of gamete transfer directly to the fallopian tubes is developed further.

With time, GIFT may come to be regarded as the modern clinical procedure that refreshed the idea that the fallopian tubes could be used to assist conception after oocyte recovery. The certainty of conception that IVF confers may thus usefully be combined with the transfer of pronuclear-stage or cleaving embryos to the tubes, either by using laparoscopy or by passing catheters into the tubes from the vagina.

References

Asch RH (1987) GIFT: International cooperative study. The first 800 cases. 5th World Congress on IVF and ET. Norfolk, Virginia 5–10 April

Asch RH, Ellsworth LR, Balmaceda JP, Wong PC (1984) Pregnancy after translaparoscopic gamete intrafallopian transfer. Lancet II:1034

Asch RH, Balmaceda JP, Ellsworth LR, Wong PC (1985) Gamete intrafallopian transfer (GIFT): a new treatment for infertility. Int J Fertil 30:41–45

Asch RH, Balmaceda JP, Ellsworth LR, Wong PC (1986a) Preliminary experiences with gamete intrafallopian transfer (GIFT). Fertil Steril 45:366–371

Asch RH, Balmaceda JP, Wong PC et al. (1986b) Gamete intrafallopian transfer (GIFT): use of minilaparotomy and an individualized regimen of induction of follicular development. Acta Eur Fertil 17:187–193

Ax RL, Ryan RJ (1979) The porcine ovarian follicle. IV. Mucopolysaccharides at different stages of development. Biol Reprod 20:1123–1132

Bize I, Driscoll D, Jackson K and McShane P (1987) pH changes during oocyte retrieval and buffering capacity of human follicular fluid. Presented at the 5th world congress on in vitro fertilization and embryo transfer. Norfolk, Virginia, 5–10 April 1987

Blackledge DG, Matson PL, Willcox DL et al. (1986) Pronuclear stage transfer and modified gamete intrafallopian transfer techniques for oligospermic cases. Med J Aust 145:173–174

Borland RM, Biggers JD, Lechene CP, Taymor ML (1980) Elemental composition of fluid in the human fallopian tube. J Reprod Fertil 58:479–482

Bourne H (1986) pH characteristics of follicular fluid and culture media. J In Vitro Fertil Embryo Transfer 3:139–140 (abstract)

Chang MC (1982) The development of in vitro fertilization from laboratory animals to human. Oxf Rev Reprod Biol 4:86–100

Chetkowski RJ, Nass TE, Matt DW et al. (1985) Optimization of hydrogen-ion concentration during aspiration of oocytes and culture and transfer of embryos. J In Vitro Fertil Embryo Transfer 2:207–212

Cohen J, Avery S, Campbell S, Mason B, Riddle A, Sharma V (1986) Follicular aspiration using a syringe suction system may damage the zona pellucida. J In Vitro Fertil Embryo Transfer 3:224–226

Corson SL, Batzer F, Eisenberg E et al. (1986) Early experience with the GIFT procedure. J Reprod Med 31:219–223

Craft I, McLeod F, Green S et al. (1982) Birth following oocyte and sperm transfer to the uterus. Lancet II:773

Craft I, Brinsden P, Simons EG (1987) How many oocytes/embryos should be transferred? Lancet II:109–110

Devroey P, Braekmans P, Smitz J et al. (1986) Pregnancy after translaparoscopic zygote intrafallopian transfer in a patient with sperm antibodies. Lancet I:1329 (letter)

Edwards RG, Steptoe PC (1983) Current status of in vitro fertilisation and implantation of human embryos. Lancet II:1265–1269

Endler GC, Stout M, Magyar DM, Hayes MF, Moghissi KS, Sacco A (1987) Uptake of anesthetic agents by follicular fluid during laparoscopic oocyte retrieval. 5th World Congress on IVF and ET. Norfolk, Virginia 5–10 April

Eppig JJ (1979) FSH stimulates hyaluronic acid synthesis by oocyte–cumulus cell complexes from mouse preovulatory follicles. Nature 281:483–484

Eppig JJ (1980) Role of serum in FSH stimulated cumulus expansion by mouse oocyte–cumulus cell complexes in vitro. Biol Reprod 22:629–633

Go KJ, Corson SL, Batzer FR, Gocial B, Eisenberg E, Huppert L (1987) Influence of CO_2 pneumoperitoneum on oocytes. 5th World Congress on IVF and ET. Norfolk, Virginia 5–10 April

Guastella G, Cefalsu E, Ciriminna R et al. (1986) One year's experience with the GIFT method. Acta Eur Fertil 17:93–97

Hayes MF, Sacco AG, Savoy-Moore RT, Magyar DM, Endler GC, Moghissi KS (1987) Anesthesia adversely affects fertilization and cleavage of human oocytes in vitro. 5th World Congress on IVF and ET Norfolk, Virginia, 5–10 April

Hinkley RE Jr, Wright BD (1985) Comparative effects of halothane, enflurane, and methoxyflurane on the incidence of abnormal development using sea urchin gametes as an in vitro model system. Anesth Analg 64:1005–1009

Hinkley RE Jr, Wright BD (1986) Effects of the volatile anesthetic halothane on fertilization and abnormal development in the sea urchin *Lytechinus variegatus*: evidence that abnormal development is due to polyspermy. Teratology 34:291–301

Hinkley RE, Wright BD, Greenberg CA (1986) Induction of the acrosome reaction in sea urchin spermatozoa by the volatile anesthetic halothane. Biol Reprod 34:119–125

Hong CY, Chaput de Saintonge DM, Turner P (1981) A simple method to measure drug effect on human sperm motility. Br J Clin Pharmacol 11:385–387

Hong CY, Wu P, Shieh CC, Chiang BN (1986) Membrane stabilising activity and inhibition of human sperm motility. Lancet II:402

Jansen RPS (1982) Spontaenous abortion incidence in the treatment of infertility (and addendum on in vitro fertilization). Am J Obstet Gynecol 143:451–473, 144:738–739

Jansen RPS (1988) Infertility and abortion. In: Huisjes HJ, Lind T (eds) Spontaneous abortion. Churchill Livingstone, Edinburgh

Jansen RPS, Anderson JC (1987) Catheterisation of the fallopian tubes from the vagina. Lancet II:309–310

Jansen RPS, Anderson JC, Radonic I, Smit J, Sutherland PD (1988a) Pregnancies after ultrasound-guided fallopian insemination with cryostored donor semen. Fertil Steril 49:179–181

Jansen RPS, Anderson JC, Sutherland PD (1988b) Non-operative embryo transfer to the fallopian tube. N Engl J Med 319:288–291

Karp L, Smith WD (1975) Experimental production of aneuploidy in mouse oocytes. Gynecol Invest 6:337–341

Lee MA, Storey BT (1986) Bicarbonate is essential for fertilization of mouse eggs: mouse sperm require it to undergo the acrosome reaction. Biol Reprod 34:349–356

Lopata A, Nayudu P, Jones G, Abramczuk J (1985) The quality of human embryos obtained by IVF. In: Testart J, Frydmann R (eds) Human in vitro fertilization. Actual problems and prospects. Elsevier, Amsterdam pp 171–186

Matson PL, Yovich JM, Junk S, Bootsma B, Yovich JL (1986) The successful recovery and fertilization of oocytes from the pouch of Douglas. J In Vitro Fertil Embryo Transfer. 3:227–230

Mazze RI, Rice SA, Wyrobek AJ, Felton JS, Brodsky JB, Baden JM (1983) Germ cell studies in mice after prolonged exposure to nitrous oxide. Toxicol Appl Pharmacol 67:370–375

McBain JC, Evans JH, Pepperell RJ, Robinson HP, Smith M, Brown JB (1980) An unexpectedly high rate of ectopic pregnancy following the induction of ovulation with human pituitary and chorionic gonadotrophin. Br J Obstet Gynaecol 87:5–9

Molloy D, Speirs AL, duPlessis Y, Gellert S, Bourne H, Johnston WIH (1986) The establishment of a successful programme of gamete intrafallopian transfer (GIFT): preliminary results. Aust NZ J Obstet Gynaecol 26:206–209

Moor RM, Crosby IM (1985) Temperature-induced abnormalities in sheep oocytes during maturation. J Reprod Fertil 75:467–473

Nakamura K, Tsunoda Y, Nagai T, Sugie T (1986) Effect of centrifugation of mouse eggs on their development in vitro and in vivo. Gamete Res 15:83–86

National Perinatal Statistics Unit and Fertility Society of Australia (1987) In vitro fertilization and GIFT pregnancies. Australia and New Zealand 1979–1986. National Perinatal Statistics Unit, Sydney; pp 38–48

Nemiro JS, McGaughey RW (1986) An alternative to in vitro fertilization embryo transfer: the successful transfer of human oocytes and spermatozoa to the distal oviduct. Fertil Steril 46:644–652

Overstreet JW, Cross NL, Morales P, Hanson FW (1987) Biology of sperm–zona pellucida interaction. 5th World Congress on IVF and ET. Norfolk, Virginia, 5–10 April

Petzelt C (1979) Biochemistry of the mitotic spindle. Int Rev Cytol 60:53–85

Puissant F, Degueldre M, Buisson L, Leroy F (1986) Effects of carbon dioxide acidification of mouse oocytes before in vitro fertilization, culture, and transfer. Gamete Res 13:223–230

Seed RF, Shakespeare TF, Muldoon MJ (1970) Carbon dioxide homeostasis during anaesthesia for laparoscopy. Anaesthesia 25:223–231

Shettles L (1979) Ova harvest with in vivo fertilization. Am J Obstet Gynecol 133:845–846

Silber S, Ord T, Borrero C, Balmaceda J, Asch R (1987) New treatment for infertility due to congenital absence of vas deferens. Lancet II:850–851 (letter)

Tesarik J, Dvorak M, Pilka L, Uher M, Soska J (1980) Die Wirkung der laparoskopischen Aspiration des Graafschen Follikels auf die Ultrastuktur von Oozyten. Zentralbl Gynakol 102:641–644

Urry RL, Jones K, Keye W, Poulson M, Worley R (1987) Prospective changes made in an in vitro fertilization program to improve pregnancy rates. 5th World Congress on IVF and ET. Norfolk, Virginia, 5–10 April

Wikland M (1987) Oocyte retrieval under the guidance of a vaginal transducer. 5th World Congress on IVF and ET. Norfolk, Virginia, 5–10 April

Yovich JL, Matson PL, Turner SR, Richardson P, Yovich JM (1986) Limitation of gamete intrafallopian transfer in the treatment of male infertility. Med J Aust 144:444

Yovich JL, Blackledge DG, Richardson PA et al. (1987) PROST for ovum donation. Lancet I:1209–1210

7 Outcome of Pregnancy

P. A. L. Lancaster

7.1 Introduction

In the period of almost a decade since the first birth after in vitro fertilization (IVF), several thousand babies have been born world-wide. However, apart from the results of the initial experience of individual IVF programmes, there are relatively few published studies with reasonable sample size that begin to answer the many questions about the outcome of IVF pregnancies.

Some of the questions requiring answers include:

1. Does the outcome of IVF pregnancies differ from those occurring after natural conceptions?
2. Are there increased risks for the mother or fetus? If so, are these risks attributable to the characteristics of the women, to the IVF procedures, to the management of IVF pregnancies, or to other factors?
3. Is fetal growth normal in IVF pregnancies?
4. Do birth defects, especially structural congenital malformations and chromosomal abnormalities, occur more commonly in infants born after IVF?

Systematic collection of data is required to provide answers to these questions. In Australia and New Zealand, evaluation of the outcome of IVF pregnancies has been enhanced by development of a voluntary register which obtains results from all IVF programmes in these two countries (Lancaster 1986). This register has several advantages: it provides results for a total population; it contains data on a much larger number of pregnancies than is obtainable within a single programme, enabling more detailed analysis of outcomes; and it avoids the tendency to publish only optimal results. This is not to say that there are no difficulties in obtaining reliable figures. Many women treated successfully by IVF continue their pregnancies in the care of referring doctors, so it is essential to obtain from them information about the outcome of pregnancy.

Unless the definitions and criteria for specific outcomes are similar for IVF and naturally conceived pregnancies (Jones et al. 1983; Lancaster 1985), comparisons between the two groups may be problematical. This should always be kept in mind in interpreting the findings of studies on the outcome of IVF pregnancies. It is usually more meaningful to exclude preclinical abortions and compare outcomes just in clinical pregnancies. Even then, ascertainment of early pregnancy losses is likely to be more complete in an IVF group followed prospectively from fertilization than in natural pregnancies.

Much of the data presented in this chapter relates to IVF pregnancies in Australia and New Zealand and is based on fertilizations in the years 1979 to 1985, thus including term births up to September 1986. All IVF programmes notify pregnancies to the register and three reports of these pregnancies have been published so far (National Perinatal Statistics Unit and Fertility Society of Australia 1984, 1985, 1987). The most recent report contained data on about 95% of pregnancies occurring in the whole period.

7.2   Characteristics of Infertile Couples

In evaluating the outcome of IVF pregnancies, it should be recalled that previously infertile women may have characteristics associated with a higher risk of adverse outcomes.

Infertile couples seeking children by IVF may have either primary or secondary infertility. While in vitro fertilization was offered initially to women with tubal causes, it has subsequently been used to treat other causes, sometimes occurring in just one partner but not uncommonly in both. In Australia and New Zealand tubal causes of infertility accounted for almost two-thirds (62.2%) of the women with pregnancies by IVF; abnormalities of sperm were the causes in 11.6%, endometriosis in 6.5%, other stated causes in 1.1%, while the cause of infertility was unexplained in 18.6%. When tubal factors are causing infertility, any risks may not be substantial if the intra-uterine environment is otherwise normal. Causes such as endometriosis, which may be accompanied by hormonal disturbances, may have different risks.

About 70% of women achieving IVF pregnancies are aged 30 or more and about 25% are at least 35, compared with 30% and 7% respectively in women giving birth in the Australian population. Also, these women may frequently have had either no previous pregnancies or poor reproductive histories.

7.3   Overall Results of IVF Pregnancies

Analysing IVF pregnancies provides an unusual situation in human reproduction because a complete fertilization cohort with known dates of fertilization can be followed to the dates of completion of the pregnancies. With natural conceptions, there have been very few studies in which the dates of fertilization were known with certainty and these studies have usually had small numbers. It is essential that, with the knowledge of outcomes at all gestational ages after fertilization, appropriate terminology is used to differentiate the various possible outcomes, especially in relation to losses in the first half of pregnancy.

There are almost no published data to provide a direct answer to the question uppermost in the minds of couples seeking treatment of their infertility by IVF, i.e. what is the likelihood of achieving a live birth for women entering an IVF programme? Results are frequently expressed in terms of the proportion of women undergoing oocyte recovery by laparoscopy, or more recently by ultrasound guidance, who subsequently progress to either successful oocyte pickup, fertilization, cleavage, embryo transfer, or ultimately pregnancy (Fishel et al. 1986). These results are rarely presented in a manner in which that important question can be answered, because women just starting treatment are usually not differentiated from those in subsequent treatment cycles.

Once a pregnancy has been achieved, there is still a considerable risk of early pregnancy loss before a final successful outcome is known. It is true that there must be many qualifying statements about the various characteristics of treated women and about the details of their treatment cycles, but the overall value of IVF in the management of infertility needs to be related to the number starting treatment. Unfortunately, it has not proved possible to answer this question with data from the register of pregnancies in Australia and New Zealand because the main emphasis has been to obtain data on the pregnancies and there is limited information so far on the number of women progressing to stages falling short of pregnancy.

As already mentioned, the various outcomes can be related to the total number of pregnancies or to clinically recognized pregnancies. In the Australian and New Zealand experience summarized in Table 7.1, 16.6% of all 1510 IVF pregnancies resulted in preclinical abortion. If these 251 preclinical abortions are then excluded from consideration, 69.0% of clinical pregnancies resulted in live birth, 23.0% in spontaneous abortion, 5.2% in ectopic pregnancy, with fewer stillbirths and therapeutic abortions.

Table 7.1. Outcome of IVF pregnancies in Australia and New Zealand

Outcome of pregnancy	Number	% of total pregnancies	% of clinical pregnancies
Preclinical abortion	251	16.6	—
Ectopic pregnancy	65	4.3	5.2
Spontaneous abortion	290	19.2	23.0
Termination of pregnancy	2	0.1	0.2
Stillbirth[a]	33	2.2	2.6
Live birth	869	57.5	69.0
Total pregnancies	1510	100.0	100.0

Source: In vitro fertilization pregnancies, Australia and New Zealand, 1979–1985.
[a] Multiple pregnancies resulting in both stillbirths and live births are included only in the stillbirth category.

The world-wide experience up to January 1984 was summarized in a report based on 1369 pregnancies (Seppala 1985). There were 285 (20.8%) preclinical abortions and spontaneous abortion occurred in 29.9% of 1084 clinical pregnancies. Ectopic pregnancy was reported in 1.8% of clinical pregnancies, but this figure was thought to be incomplete. Several groups in the United Kingdom, the United States and France have also reported results based on at least 100 pregnancies.

Relatively few pregnancies have occurred after the use of donor gametes, donor embryos or frozen embryos. The early experience suggests that the outcome of these pregnancies is similar to that of other IVF pregnancies.

Maternal age is an important risk factor in determining the outcome of pregnancy. As shown in Table 7.2, live births were more likely in women aged less than 35 than in older women. This is due to the increasing risk of spontaneous abortion and ectopic pregnancy (except in the youngest age group with small numbers) in the more advanced maternal age groups.

Table 7.2. Maternal age and outcome of pregnancy

Outcome of pregnancy	Maternal age (years)					
	<25	25–29	30–34	35–39	40+	Total[a]
Preclinical abortion	9	72	101	61	5	251
Ectopic pregnancy (%)[b]	4 (12.9)	15 (4.3)	24 (4.2)	20 (7.0)	2 (10.0)	65 (5.2)
Spontaneous abortion (%)[c]	4 (14.8)	72 (21.8)	116 (21.0)	89 (33.8)	8 (44.4)	290 (24.3)
Stillbirth	2	11	18	1	—	33
Live birth (%)[d]	21 (67.7)	247 (71.6)	418 (72.4)	173 (60.9)	10 (50.0)	869 (69.0)
Total pregnancies	40	417	678[e]	345[e]	25	1510

Source: In vitro fertilization pregnancies, Australia and New Zealand, 1979–1985.
[a] Total includes 5 pregnancies in which maternal age was not stated.
[b] % of clinical pregnancies.
[c] % of intra-uterine pregnancies.
[d] % of clinical pregnancies.
[e] % Total includes 1 termination of pregnancy.

The outcome of pregnancy may also be influenced by some aspects of treatment, especially the number of embryos transferred to the mother (Table 7.3). In these data, live births occurred most frequently after transfer of four embryos; transfer of two or three embryos was also associated with a better outcome than transfer of one or five embryos. The likelihood of achieving live births after IVF in selected groups of women is a function both of the pregnancy rate and of the proportion of live births occurring in these pregnancies.

Table 7.3. Number of embryos transferred and outcome of clinical pregnancies

Outcome of pregnancy	Number of embryos transferred					
	One	Two	Three	Four	Five	Total[a]
Preclinical abortion	38	75	68	58	12	251
Ectopic pregnancy (%)[b]	8 (5.0)	17 (5.2)	26 (5.9)	8 (3.0)	4 (11.1)	65 (5.2)
Spontaneous abortion (%)[b]	47 (29.2)	80 (24.4)	102 (23.3)	41 (15.3)	9 (25.0)	290 (23.0)
Stillbirth (%)[b]	5 (3.1)	5 (1.5)	13 (3.0)	10 (3.7)	—	33 (2.6)
Live birth (%)[b]	100 (62.1)	226 (68.9)	296 (67.7)	208 (77.6)	23 (63.9)	869 (69.0)
Total pregnancies	199[c]	403	505	326[c]	48	1510

Source: In vitro fertilization pregnancies, Australia and New Zealand, 1979–1985.
[a] Total includes 3 pregnancies with six embryos transferred and 26 pregnancies in which the number of embryos was not stated.
[b] % of clinical pregnancies.
[c] Total includes 1 termination of pregnancy.

Women who decide to attempt more than one IVF pregnancy are more likely to achieve a successful outcome in the second pregnancy than in the first. In the Australian and New Zealand experience of 1510 pregnancies, 115 (7.6%) were repeat pregnancies. In the first pregnancy, 11.4% had a live birth, but this improved to 64.8% in the second pregnancy.

7.4 Early Pregnancy Losses

7.4.1 Preclinical Abortion

The diagnosis of preclinical abortion is based on a serum level of human chorionic gonadotrophin (hCG) within the range usually detected in a normal pregnancy. However, the levels of hCG are not sustained for more than a few weeks after implantation and there is no clinical evidence that pregnancy has occurred.

In their initial series of more than 200 pregnancies, Edwards and Steptoe (1983) reported an incidence of preclinical abortion (or biochemical pregnancy) of 13.4%. In the large Australian and New Zealand experience (Table 7.1), preclinical abortion occurred in 16.6% of 1510 pregnancies. This figure probably underestimated its real incidence because testing for these pregnancies in some IVF programmes has become less stringent than it was previously. In contrast to the pattern seen in spontaneous abortion, there was no clear-cut association between preclinical abortion and maternal age (Table 7.2), possibly indicating that the quality of the embryo may be more important than maternal factors in the failure of the pregnancy. Recent studies of chromosomal abnormalities in oocytes recovered during stimulated cycles in patients with infertility (Wramsby et al. 1987), and in pre-implantation embryos obtained after fertilization in vitro (Angell et al. 1986), offer possible explanations for these early embryonic losses.

7.4.2 Spontaneous Abortion

Clinical spontaneous abortions of less than 20 weeks' gestation occur in about one-quarter to one-third of IVF pregnancies (Australian In Vitro Fertilisation Collaborative Group 1985; Steptoe 1985). Because IVF pregnancies can be followed prospectively from the time of fertilization until completion of the pregnancy, ascertainment of spontaneous abortion is probably better than in natural conceptions. Nevertheless, the occurrence of spontaneous abortion is considerably more common in IVF pregnancies than the usual incidence of about 10%–15%. The older ages of women achieving IVF pregnancies is certainly a factor. If only intra-uterine clinical pregnancies are considered, there was a threefold difference in the incidence of spontaneous abortion between the youngest (less than 25) and oldest (40 and over) maternal age groups (Table 7.2). The overall incidence in this series was 24.3%. More than three-quarters of these spontaneous abortions occurred before a gestational age of 12 weeks.

While there have been substantial numbers of case reports of chromosomal abnormalities in spontaneous abortions after IVF (Seppala 1985), there have been no systematic studies to determine what proportion of these abortions is due to such abnormalities.

7.4.3 Ectopic Pregnancy

Ectopic pregnancies occur in about 1% of natural conceptions and several studies have shown an increasing incidence (Budnick and Pakter 1982; Shiono et al. 1982). The incidence in IVF pregnancies is from about 2 to 5 times higher (Ausralian In Vitro Fertilisation Collaborative Group 1985; Seppala 1985; Frydman et al. 1986; Andrews et al. 1986), although Steptoe (1985) reported only 4 ectopic pregnancies in his series of 365 IVF pregnancies.

Our most recent report of IVF pregnancies (Table 7.1) showed 65 (5.2%) ectopic pregnancies among 1259 clinical pregnancies. Women aged less than 25, or 35 and over, had higher rates than those aged 25–34. Ectopic pregnancy was more likely to occur with tubal causes than with other causes of infertility. There was no clear-cut association between ectopic pregnancy and the number of embryos transferred to the uterus (Table 7.3). In one study of 10 ectopic pregnancies (Martinez and Trounson 1986), no major predisposing factor was identified. On the other hand, Yovich et al. (1985) concluded that embryo transfer to the uterine fundus was more likely to be associated with ectopic pregnancy than transfer to a midcavity position. Other factors possibly contributing to this higher incidence of ectopic pregnancy include the tubal disease – and frequently tubal surgery – that has caused infertility, and the volume and rate of injection of fluid at embryo transfer (Leeton 1982).

Numerous cases of combined ectopic and intra-uterine pregnancies have now been reported following transfer of multiple embryos. In some instances, the intra-uterine pregnancy progressed to a live birth after surgical treatment of the ectopic pregnancy. Other variants of ectopic pregnancy have included twin tubal pregnancies and ovarian pregnancies. Further study of the site of IVF and natural tubal pregnancies may give a better indication of possible causes.

7.5 Viable Pregnancies

7.5.1 Duration of Pregnancy

The reports from the register of IVF pregnancies in Australia and New Zealand have consistently shown a high incidence of preterm delivery in pregnancies of at least 20 weeks' gestation (National Perinatal Statistics Unit and Fertility Society of Australia 1984, 1985, 1987; Australian In Vitro Fertilisation Collaborative Group 1985). In 890 pregnancies with stated dates of fertilization and birth (Table 7.4), delivery occurred before 37 weeks in 240 (27.0%). Multiple pregnancy due to transfer of more than one embryo was an important factor but, even in single pregnancies, preterm birth occurred in 18.5%, about three times more commonly than in natural pregnancies.

Table 7.4.   Duration of single and multiple pregnancies[a] (percentages in brackets)

Gestational age (weeks)	Single	Twin	Triplet	Total[b]
20–27	8 (1.2)	8 (4.8)	1 (3.2)	17 (1.9)
28–31	16 (2.3)	10 (6.0)	11 (35.5)	37 (4.2)
32–36	104 (15.1)	63 (37.7)	18 (58.1)	186 (20.9)
37–41	558 (80.8)	85 (50.9)	1 (3.2)	644 (72.4)
42 or more	5 (0.7)	1 (0.6)	—	6 (0.7)
Total	691 (100)	167 (100)	31 (100)	890 (100)

Source: In vitro fertilization pregnancies, Australia and New Zealand, 1979–1985.
[a] Table excludes 12 pregnancies with unstated gestational age.
[b] Total includes 1 quadruplet pregnancy of 34 weeks' gestation.

The experience of several other groups, based on small numbers of pregnancies in single IVF units, has not shown a similar high incidence of preterm birth but its definition was not always clearly stated. Frydman et al. (1986) reported premature delivery in 6.3% of single pregnancies, while Andrews and colleagues (1986) found that 8% of deliveries occurred before 36 weeks' gestation.

The reasons for the high incidence of preterm delivery in single births – at least in Australia and New Zealand – are uncertain. Maternal age and the cause of infertility do not seem to be important factors (National Perinatal Statistics Unit and Fertility Society of Australia 1987). Very few published studies have examined obstetric complications (see Sect. 7.5.3), but bleeding in pregnancy occurred frequently in one study (Andrews et al, 1986). Elective intervention, either by induction of labour or Caesarean section, may be more common than usual, but appropriate studies have not been done. Abnormal placentation and infection associated with the procedures of IVF are other less likely possibilities.

7.5.2   Multiple Pregnancy

Multiple births are very common after IVF due to the frequent transfer of more than one embryo. Among 902 pregnancies of at least 20 weeks' gestation in Australia and New Zealand, there were 202 (22.4%) multiple pregnancies including 169 twin pregnancies, 32 sets of triplets and 1 set of quadruplets. About 1% of natural conceptions result in multiple pregnancy. Other groups have reported fewer multiple pregnancies, presumably because they transfer fewer embryos. In the world-wide series of confinements up to January 1984, 12.6% were multiple births (Seppala 1985). The influence of the number of embryos transferred is clearly shown in Table 7.5. Multiple pregnancy occurred in more than 30% of pregnancies in which three or four embryos had been transferred. While most multiple pregnancies after IVF are due to transfer of multiple embryos, monozygotic twins have also been reported (Mettler et al. 1984; Yovich et al. 1984).

Not all multiple pregnancies are still evident by the second half of pregnancy. The number of gestational sacs is usually assessed by ultrasound in the early stages of an IVF pregnancy. About 40% of implantation sites have been shown to disappear (Jones 1986); histological confirmation has been made in one case by examination of the placenta (Sulak and Dobson 1986).

Table 7.5. Number of embryos transferred and multiple pregnancies[a] (percentages in brackets)

Number of embryos transferred	Single	Twin	Triplet	Total
One	104 (99.0)	1 (1.0)	—	105 (100)
Two	204 (88.3)	27 (11.7)	—	231 (100)
Three	208 (67.3)	84 (27.2)	17 (5.5)	309 (100)
Four	151 (69.3)	52 (23.9)	14 (6.4)	218[b] (100)
Five	20 (87.0)	3 (13.0)	—	23 (100)
Six	1 (50.0)	1 (50.0)	—	2 (100)
Total	688 (77.6)	168 (18.7)	31 (3.5)	888[b] (100)

Source: In vitro fertilization pregnancies, Australia and New Zealand, 1979–1985.
[a] Table excludes 14 pregnancies with unstated number of embryos.
[b] Includes 1 quadruplet pregnancy.

There remains a dilemma in deciding how many embryos should be transferred to the mother. Transfer of more than one embryo results in higher pregnancy rates (Wood et al. 1984; Steptoe 1985). Also, our data show that live births are most likely in those pregnancies in which four embryos are transferred (Table 7.3). These apparent advantages must be weighed against the greater risks of fetal and neonatal death in multiple pregnancies (see Sect. 7.6.4).

7.5.3 Obstetric Complications

Very few studies of the course of IVF pregnancies and their complications have been published so far. Andrews et al. (1986) reported vaginal bleeding during pregnancy in 59% of 91 IVF pregnancies, mainly in the first trimester. Bleeding was sometimes associated with early fetal loss in multiple pregnancies. Complete or marginal placenta praevia occurred in two cases.

Frydman et al. (1986) compared the course of 79 singleton IVF pregnancies with 142 pregnancies which followed induced ovulation and 3841 naturally conceived pregnancies within the same hospital. Bleeding in the first trimester was slightly more common in the IVF group and maternal hypertension occurred twice as often, but a higher proportion of IVF patients were primigravid. No abnormality was detected in 52 placentas that were examined histologically. Breech presentations were also more common in the IVF group.

7.5.4 Mode of Delivery

Most reported series of IVF pregnancies show Caesarean birth rates well in excess of those found in confinements following natural conception. In Australia and New Zealand (National Perinatal Statistics Unit and Fertility Society of Australia 1987), delivery by Caesarean section occurred in 43.9% of all IVF confinements. This rate was 39.3% for single births, 54.3% for twins, and 86.7% for triplets.

The overall Caesarean birth rate reported by 65 groups up to January 1984 was 49% (Seppala 1985). Similar rates were reported by other groups: 56% in England (Steptoe 1985, p. 248), 58% in the United States (Andrews et al. 1986) and 47% in France (Frydman et al. 1986).

Factors contributing to these high Caesarean birth rates include advanced maternal age in IVF pregnancies, the history of prolonged infertility, sometimes poor reproductive histories, multiple pregnancy, and breech presentations in preterm confinements. Undoubtedly many obstetricians managing the pregnancies of women who have had difficulty in conceiving elect to perform a Caesarean section because of anxiety about the outcome of the IVF pregnancy.

7.6 Infants Born After In Vitro Fertilization

7.6.1 Sex Ratio

The data in Table 7.6 show the sex ratio of 1104 births in Australia and New Zealand. The overall male to female ratio of 1.06:1.00 was similar to population figures. In single births, there were almost equal numbers of males and females; in twins, there were more males than females, while there were more females than males among the triplets. Relatively small numbers probably account for the variations observed in multiple births.

Table 7.6. Sex of infants in single and multiple births

Plurality	Male	Female	Sex ratio (M : F)
Single	338	339	1.00 : 1.00
Twins	183	150	1.22 : 1.00
Triplets	42	48	0.88 : 1.00
Quadruplets	4	—	—
Total	567	537	1.06 : 1.00

Source: In vitro fertilization pregnancies, Australia and New Zealand, 1979–1985.

Among 524 infants reported from IVF groups around the world (Seppala 1985), there were 264 males and 260 females. The sex ratio in another large series of 284 births was 0.95:1.00 (Steptoe 1985, p. 248).

Although early results based on small numbers of births suggested a possible excess of girls born after IVF, these reports were not substantiated by subsequent findings.

7.6.2 Birthweight

The birthweights of 1102 live and stillborn infants are given in Table 7.7. The incidence of low birthweight (less than 2500 g) was 34. 8%, more than five times higher than the population figure of about 6%. Multiple births were an important factor with an incidence of low birthweight of 57.1% in twins and 95.5% in triplets. Nevertheless, even in single IVF births, the incidence of low birthweight was 15.5%. This high incidence of low birthweight was associated with frequent preterm delivery (see Sect. 7.5.1). Fetal growth retardation did not appear to be a factor (see Sect. 7.6.3).

Table 7.7. Birthweight of infants in single and multiple births[a] (percentages in brackets)

Birthweight (g)	Single	Twin	Triplet	Total[b]
Less than 500	—	2 (0.6)	3 (3.4)	5 (0.5)
500–999	12 (1.8)	14 (4.2)	2 (2.2)	28 (2.5)
1000–1499	20 (3.0)	27 (8.1)	27 (30.3)	74 (6.7)
1500–1999	19 (2.8)	33 (9.9)	34 (38.2)	88 (8.0)
2000–2499	54 (8.0)	114 (34.2)	19 (21.3)	189 (17.2)
2500–2999	142 (21.0)	107 (32.1)	4 (4.5)	253 (23.0)
3000–3499	252 (37.3)	34 (10.2)	—	286 (26.0)
3500–3999	133 (19.7)	1 (0.3)	—	134 (12.2)
4000 or more	44 (6.5)	1 (0.3)	—	45 (4.1)
Total	676 (100)	333 (100)	89 (100)	1102 (100)

Source: In vitro fertilization pregnancies, Australia and New Zealand, 1979–1985.
[a] Table excludes 36 infants with unstated birthweight.
[b] Includes 4 infants from quadruplet pregnancy.

In their study comparing IVF and other births in the same hospital, Frydman et al. (1986) found that the mean birthweight of 79 IVF infants was similar to that of the other infants and slightly higher than infants born after induced ovulation.

7.6.3 Fetal Growth

In Table 7.8, the birthweight of 969 liveborn IVF infants in Australia and New Zealand are compared with birthweight for gestational age percentiles of an Australian hospital population (Kitchen 1968). Because of small numbers of markedly preterm infants, only IVF infants of at least 32 weeks' gestation were included.

Table 7.8. Birthweight percentiles of liveborn infants in single and multiple births (percentages in brackets)

Birthweight percentile	Single	Twin	Triplet	Total
Less than 5th	15 (2.4)	17 (5.9)	6 (12)	38 (3.9)
5th to <10th	16 (2.5)	15 (5.2)	1 (2)	32 (3.3)
10th to <25th	92 (14.5)	65 (22.7)	12 (24)	169 (17.4)
25th to <50th	184 (29.1)	124 (43.4)	17 (34)	325 (33.5)
50th to <75th	171 (27.0)	53 (18.5)	12 (24)	236 (24.4)
75th to <90th	99 (15.6)	10 (3.5)	2 (4)	111 (11.5)
90th to <95th	32 (5.1)	2 (0.7)	—	34 (3.5)
95th or more	24 (3.8)	—	—	24 (2.5)
Total infants	633 (100)	286 (100)	50 (100)	969 (100)

Source: In vitro fertilization pregnancies, Australia and New Zealand, 1979–1985.

These data, and a similar study of 85 singleton infants in the United States (Andrews et al. 1986), do not provide any evidence of fetal growth retardation after IVF. The percentages given in brackets show that, for single births, the proportion of infants within each percentile range was comparable to that expected. Fetal growth retardation is common in multiple pregnancy, so it is not surprising that relatively more of these infants were found to have birthweights within the lower percentile range.

7.6.4   Perinatal Mortality

The high incidence of preterm delivery and low birthweight after IVF increases the risk of perinatal death. Table 7.9 shows an overall perinatal death rate of 47.5 per 1000 births among fetuses and infants of at least 20 weeks' gestation. This is about four times higher than in the Australian population. After adjusting for maternal age differences, the observed number of perinatal deaths was still about twice the expected number. Fetal death rates in both single and multiple pregnancies were about three times higher than neonatal death rates.

Table 7.9.   Perinatal deaths[a]

Outcome	Single	Multiple	Total
Fetal deaths			
Number	17	24	41
Rate per 1000 births	24.3	54.8	36.0
Neonatal deaths			
Number	6	7	13
Rate per 1000 live births	8.8	16.9	11.9
Perinatal deaths			
Number[b]	23 (7.9)	31 (19.7)	54 (27.6)
Rate per 1000 total births	32.9	70.8	47.5

Source: In vitro fertilization pregnancies, Australia and New Zealand, 1979–1985.
[a] Numbers and rates based on 1097 live births and 41 fetal deaths of at least 20 weeks' gestation.
[b] Figures in brackets give expected numbers after adjusting for maternal age differences between IVF births and Australian population.

Preterm delivery of low birthweight infants is probably the main reason for the excess of neonatal deaths, but the factors resulting in the higher fetal death rate have yet to be determined. Eight perinatal deaths, including 6 fetal deaths, occurred in infants with major congenital malformations.

7.6.5   Congenital Malformations

Several authors have reviewed the factors that could lead to a greater risk of congenital malformations after IVF (Schlesselmann 1979; Biggers 1981; Lancaster 1985). These factors include the more advanced ages of infertile couples, increasing the risk of chromosomal abnormalities and point mutations; the underlying causes of infertility and the drugs used to induce ovulation or for luteal phase support; and the procedures of IVF, possibly resulting in polyspermy, delayed fertilization of oocytes, and freezing and thawing of embryos. It has also been suggested that favourable laboratory conditions in IVF may even reduce the risks of abnormal embryos (Jones et al. 1983).

Among 1138 births in Australia and New Zealand, major congenital malformations or chromosomal abnormalities were reported in 26 (2.3%). These included three pregnancies in which therapeutic abortion was performed at 17, 20 and 22 weeks respectively, following prenatal diagnosis of fetuses with duplication of part of the short arm of chromosome 7, osteogenesis imperfecta, and XYY syndrome. In the case of the fetus with osteogenesis imperfecta, the embryo had been frozen. Table 7.10 shows the incidence of non-chromosomal and chromosomal abnormalities in each maternal age group. No specific pattern of birth defects was noted in these fetuses and infants.

Table 7.10. Congenital malformations[a] by maternal age

Maternal age	Total births	Non-chromosomal	Chromosomal	Total
Less than 25	31	—	—	—
25–29	334	3	—	3
30–34	560	10	1	11
35–39	202	7	2	9
40 or more	10	1	2	3
All ages	1138[b]	21	5	26

Source: In vitro fertilization pregnancies, Australia and New Zealand, 1979–1985.
[a] Includes 3 terminations of pregnancy after prenatal diagnosis.
[b] Includes 1 with unstated maternal age.

Although the overall incidence of 2.3% was slightly higher than the Australian population incidence of 1.5% (National Perinatal Statistics Unit 1986), these rates are not directly comparable because the methods of ascertainment of cases differ. Population figures on therapeutic abortions are less complete than those for IVF pregnancies and notification of births in the latter group may be better. The number of births reported by other IVF groups has been too small to give meaningful rates and information about the outcome of pregnancies has not always been available. Chromosomal abnormalities have been found in spontaneously aborted fetuses, but no systematic studies have been reported.

While the number of IVF births is still too small to give conclusive evidence that IVF does not cause an increased risk of congenital malformations, any risk appears to be small. These findings suggest that routine amniocentesis in IVF pregnancies is not necessary unless the usual indications, such as advanced maternal age, are present.

7.6.6 Follow-up Studies

There have been no published studies in which developmental and psychological assessments of children born after IVF have been compared with a suitable control group. The high incidence of preterm delivery and low birthweight reported in IVF births (Tables 7.4 and 7.7) emphasizes the importance of selecting appropriate controls in these follow-up studies.

Two small studies (Mushin et al. 1985, 1986; Yovich et al. 1986), based on assessments of 49 and 20 children respectively, did not indicate any specific problems that could be attributed to IVF. Several studies in Australia, the United Kingdom and the United States are in progress.

7.7 Conclusions

Results from a population-based register of IVF pregnancies, and from other studies in single IVF programmes, show that ectopic pregnancy, and probably also spontaneous abortion, occur more commonly in IVF than in naturally conceived pregnancies.

Obstetric complications after IVF have not been adequately studied. Bleeding in early pregnancy, possibly related to embryonic loss in multiple pregnancy in some cases, may be more common than usual. Other complications such as hypertension may reflect maternal risk factors.

There is a high incidence of preterm delivery and low birthweight in IVF pregnancies, partly attributable to the frequent occurrence of multiple births. These outcomes contribute to the increased risk of perinatal death in IVF pregnancies.

Fetal growth appears to be normal in IVF pregnancies. The sex ratio and the incidence at birth of major congenital malformations and chromosomal abnormalities are similar to those found in natural conceptions.

Further studies of the outcome of IVF pregnancies are required to confirm these findings and to determine possible causes of adverse outcomes. Follow-up studies of children born after IVF, and of appropriate control groups, are also needed.

Acknowledgements

I thank the staff of IVF units in Australia and New Zealand for providing their data to the IVF register and also the staff of the National Perinatal Statistics Unit for their assistance in data processing and preparation of the manuscript. The National Perinatal Statistics Unit is funded by a grant from the Australian Institute of Health.

References

Andrews MC, Muasher SJ, Levy DL et al. (1986) An analysis of the obstetric outcome of 125 consecutive pregnancies conceived in vitro and resulting in 100 deliveries. Am J Obstet Gynecol 154:848–854

Angell RR, Templeton AA, Aitken RJ (1986) Chromosome studies in human in vitro fertilization. Hum Genet 72:333–339

Australian In Vitro Fertilisation Collaborative Group (1985) High incidence of preterm births and early losses in pregnancy after in vitro fertilisation. Br Med J 291:1160–1163

Biggers JD (1981) In vitro fertilization and embryo transfer in human beings. N Engl J Med 304:336–342

Budnick LD, Pakter J (1982) Ectopic pregnancy in New York City, 1975–1980. Am J Public Health 72:580–584

Edwards RG, Steptoe PC (1983) Current status of in-vitro fertilisation and implantation of human embryos. Lancet II:1265–1269

Fishel S, Webster J, Jackson P, Faratian B (1986) Presentation of information on in-vitro fertilisation. Lancet I:1444 (letter)

Frydman R, Belaisch-Allart J, Fries N et al. (1986) An obstetric assessment of the first 100 births from the in vitro fertilization program at Clamart, France. Am J Obstet Gynecol 154:550–555

Jones HW Jr (1986) The impact of in vitro fertilization on the practice of gynecology and obstetrics. Int J Fertil 31:99, 102–105, 109–111

Jones HW Jr, Acosta AA, Andrews MC et al. (1983) What is a pregnancy? A question for programs of in vitro fertilization. Fertil Steril 40:728–733

Kitchen WH (1968) The relationship between birth weight and gestational age in an Australian hospital population. Aust Paediatr J 4:29–37

Lancaster PAL (1985) Obstetric outcome. Clin Obstet Gynaecol 12:847–864

Lancaster PAL (1986) Health registers for congenital malformations and in-vitro fertilization. Clin Reprod Fertil 4:27–37

Leeton JF (1982) Discussion on the laparoscopic recovery of oocytes. In: Edwards RG, Purdy JM (eds) Human conception in vitro. Academic Press, London, p 128

Martinez F, Trounson A (1986) An analysis of factors associated with ectopic pregnancy in a human in vitro fertilization program. Fertil Steril 45:79–87

Mettler L, Grillo M, Riedel H-H, Michelmann HW, Semm K (1984) Multiple pregnancies after in vitro fertilization and embryo replacement. J In Vitro Fertil Embryo Transfer 1:26

Mushin D, Spensley J, Barreda-Hanson M (1985) Children of IVF. Clin Obstet Gynaecol 12:865–876

Mushin DN, Barreda-Hanson MC, Spensley JC (1986) In vitro fertilization children: early psychosocial development. J In Vitro Fertil Embryo Transfer 3:247–252

National Perinatal Statistics Unit (1986) Congenital malformations, Australia, 1981–1984. National Perinatal Statistics Unit, Sydney

National Perinatal Statistics Unit, Fertility Society of Australia (1984) In vitro fertilization pregnancies, Australia, 1980–1983. National Perinatal Statistics Unit, Sydney

National Perinatal Statistics Unit, Fertility Society of Australia (1985) In vitro fertilization pregnancies, Australia and New Zealand, 1979–1984. National Perinatal Statistics Unit, Sydney

National Perinatal Statistics Unit, Fertility Society of Australia (1987) In vitro fertilization pregnancies, Australia and New Zealand, 1979–1985. National Perinatal Statistics Unit, Sydney

Schlesselmann JJ (1979) How does one assess the risk of abnormalities from human in vitro fertilization? Am J Obstet Gynecol 135:135–148

Seppala M (1985) The world collaborative report on in vitro fertilization and embryo replacement: current state of the art in January 1984. Ann NY Acad Sci 442:558–563

Shiono PH, Harlap S, Pellegrin F (1982) Ectopic pregnancies: rising incidence rates in Northern California. Am J Public Health 72:173–175

Steptoe PC (1985) Studies in pregnancy established by in vitro fertilisation. In: Thompson W, Joyce DN, Newton JR (eds) In vitro fertilisation and donor insemination. The Royal College of Obstetricians and Gynaecologists, London, pp 241–251

Sulak LE, Dobson MG (1986) The vanishing twin: pathologic confirmation of an ultrasonographic phenomenon. Obstet Gynecol 68:811–815

Wood C, Downing B, Trounson A, Rogers P (1984) Clinical implications of developments in in vitro fertilisation. Br Med J 289:978–980

Wramsby H, Fredga K, Liedholm P (1987) Chromosome analysis of human oocytes recovered from preovulatory follicles in stimulated cycles. N Eng J Med 316: 121–124

Yovich JL, Stanger JD, Grauaug A et al. (1984) Monozygotic twins from in vitro fertilization. Fertil Steril 41:833–837

Yovich JL, Turner SR, Murphy AJ (1985) Embryo transfer technique as a cause of ectopic pregnancies in in vitro fertilization. Fertil Steril 44:318–321

Yovich JL, Parry TS, French NP, Grauaug AA (1986) Developmental assessment of twenty in vitro fertilization (IVF) infants at their first birthday. J In Vitro Fertil Embryo Transfer 3:253–257

8 Androlgy, Male Factor Infertility and IVF

C. A. Yates, Caroline Thomas, G. T. Kovacs and D. M. de Kretser

8.1 Introduction

This chapter deals with the methods for obtaining motile sperm from the semen sample for insemination of the female partner's oocytes, particularly in cases of male factor infertility, and, briefly, with the assessment of the male partner prior to an IVF cycle. Due to the comparative ease of obtaining the male gametes, compared with the female's, many basic diagnostic tests and treatments which could improve the chances of optimal fertilization may be disregarded. This chapter will also outline the basic steps required to ensure that the male partner is fully investigated.

8.2 Assessment of the Male

It is important that the male partner in a couple entering an IVF programme is thoroughly investigated to determine the existence of any problem that may effect his fertility. One of the earliest steps used to investigate the fertility status of a couple is the assessment of several semen analyses at a reputable laboratory with experienced semen analysis technicians, i.e. a laboratory which follows the protocols described in the World Health Organization's (WHO) *Laboratory manual for the examination of human semen and semen–cervical mucus interaction* (1987). Many of the methods described briefly in the following sections are well documented in this manual. It is important to note that several semen analyses should be carried out, as the variation in semen parameters between semen analyses is common and is well documented (Baker et al. 1981; Tjoa et al. 1982; Poland et al. 1985). Any problems detected in the semen analysis should be investigated further to determine whether treatment can improve semen quality.

8.2.1 Semen Analysis

The standard semen analysis should contain information about the number of spermatozoa, motility, morphology and viability together with an assessment of whether leucocytes are present. The methods used for a semen analysis should follow, at the very least, the guidelines set out in the WHO laboratory manual (1987). Another excellent guide for a semen laboratory is given by Mortimer (1985), which covers all details of the required protocols.

Briefly, the semen analysis is performed on specimens collected by masturbation or, if there is difficulty in producing the sample, in a silastic semen collection device which can be worn during coitus (Zavos 1985a, b). The sample should be collected after at least 3 days' abstinence from ejaculation. The general appearance of the semen sample should be noted, as any abnormal colour or odour may be indicative of infection. The sample should be viewed microscopically after liquefaction, with the amount of cellular debris and sperm agglutination recorded, usually by a grading system. The percentage motility is then assessed, and some variation between laboratories exists in the techniques used for this parameter. At least 200 sperm are counted, and each sperm viewed is classified as being motile or non-motile. If motile, the sperm should then be defined as having either progressive or non-progressive motility (Eliasson 1971). This can be taken further and the sperm graded on a subjective assessment of the speed of the sperm. From these observations the percentage of progressive motility can be calculated subjectively and then the motility index, a figure which represents the extent of the forward progressiveness of the sperm within the sample. The number which is of importance within an IVF system is the percentage of progressively motile sperm.

The sperm concentration is measured by taking an aliquot from the semen sample which has been agitated while undergoing liquefaction. The sperm are diluted and immobilized in either tap water or a weak fixative. The diluted sample is then placed in a haemocytometer and then counted and the concentration per millilitre calculated. There are chambers available which have been specifically designed for semen analyses, such as the Makler chamber or the Horvell fertility chamber. These can be used with fresh undiluted samples and can be used for the calculation of both the concentration and the motility.

Sperm morphology is examined on a stained smear. There are various stains suitable, with the Papanicolaou or the Bryan–Leishman staining methods (WHO 1987) predominating. A quick method for assessing morphology is the use of pre-stained Testsimplets which stain the sperm in the manner of the Papanicolaou method within 15–30 minutes. The sperm should then be classified as being normal or abnormal and, if abnormal, further classified into various subgroups of abnormalities. Leucocytes can be identified if the Bryan–Leishman stain is used. However, identification is preferable and more rapid using a peroxidase staining method which allows the differentiation of the leucocytes from other forms of cellular debris. The leucocytes should be counted on a haemocytometer (or one of the specific semen analysis chambers) after staining and expressed as a concentration per millilitre. Finally, the percentage of alive sperm can be obtained by the use of a dye exclusion test. An aliquot of the semen sample is mixed with an equal volume of 0.5% of either eosin yellow or blue in phosphate buffered saline and viewed microscopically as a wet mount.

An important test that should be carried out during the initial investigation of a couple's infertility is for the presence of sperm antibodies in both the male and the female. In the male, there are various tests available but the immunobead test (Clarke et al. 1985) is the simplest and only requires the semen sample for testing. The immunobeads are microscopic beads which are covered with either anti-human IgG or IgA. These are washed and mixed with the semen sample and the percentage binding to various sections of the spermatozoa are recorded. The immunobeads test by itself, however, is not a significant test for IVF. It has to be associated with a mucus penetration test to enable conclusions to be made. If the spermatozoa are found to bind the immunobeads significantly and are also unable to penetrate cervical mucus, then the chances of fertilization are reduced.

This is just a brief overview of the basic semen analysis methods which should be used. As mentioned previously, there are excellent manuals available which give thorough protocols on each of the tests described.

8.2.2 Advanced Semen Analysis

This section covers tests which are not part of the standard semen analysis – that is, they are tests that need not be performed on every semen sample. Only a general review is given for each of these tests as they are intricate and the exact methods required go beyond the auspices of this review. Many of these tests have also yet to prove whether they are, in fact, related to fertility in vitro.

8.2.2.1 Objective Measurement of Motility

The objective measurement of motility has long been regarded as important in the analysis of the semen sample. Also, the simple measurement of sperm movement characteristics, such as lateral head amplitude, velocity, straight-line velocity and head rotation, have also been desired measurement parameters as these are thought to have some relationship to the fertilizing potential of the semen sample. There have been various exotic methods used, such as turbimetric analysis and spectrophotometric methods (Timouran and Watchmaker 1970; Atherton 1970). However, it has only been since the recent development of computer systems, which are able to digitize and then analyse the image of the motile sperm, that extensive subjective measurement has been possible. One simple yet effective method is to utilize time-lapse photography of spermatozoa and then determine the motility characteristics from the sperm tracks (Janick and MacLeod 1970; Overstreet et al. 1979; Aitken et al. 1982, 1985; Mortimer 1986). A variation of this is the multiple exposure method (MEP) where the sperm are photographed over a set period of time, usually in the region of 1 second, and the sperm illuminated by a stroboscopic attachment which allows six multiple exposures of the field over the time period. The photograph can then be printed and the distance the sperm travels measured and the velocity calculated (Makler 1978, 1979, 1980; Makler et al. 1979; Milligan et al. 1980; Kamindono et al. 1982, 1984). The introduction of computers has allowed the refinement of this technique, whereby the photograph or a projection of the photograph can be viewed on a digitizing board and the sperm traced with a digitizing pen. The computer system then ascertains which sperm are motile and non-motile and for the motile sperm, the velocities and straight-line velocities can be calculated (Makler et al. 1980; Cohen et al. 1982a).

Another method which allows the measurement of sperm motility is that of Katz and Overstreet (1981) which makes use of a system whereby various fields are videotaped and then played back, during which an individual sperm is tracked by means of an overlay on the screen. This method allows the sperm straight-line velocity to be calculated and it has been shown to compare well with the subjective semen analysis system (Jenks et al. 1982). An advancement of this technique is described by Holt et al. (1985) where the video image of the sperm is played back through a computer system and the sperm are tracked manually on the computer screen; the analysis of the track is then carried out by the computer. Of course, the main desire has been to work towards a fully automatic system using image analysis. This has been achieved initially by filming and then tracking the sperm with the computer (Katz and Dott 1975; Liu and Warme 1977; Amann and Hammerstedt 1980). Recently there has been the introduction of commercially available semen analysis systems which can analyse the sperm in real time and can be carried out on either fresh or videotaped samples.

8.2.2.2 Sperm Transport

The assessment of sperm transport leads on from sperm movement characteristics in playing a major part in how the sperm is able to reach the oocyte in vivo. The movement characteristics that allow movement through the female reproductive tract are also thought to play a major part in the penetration of the zona pellucida and, finally, into the vestments of the oocyte. The post-coital test (PCT) has been used to predict the success of IVF. Unfortunately there are conflicting results on this matter, with a correlation found between the PCT results and subsequent success in IVF by one group. However, Cohen et al. (1984b) and Matson et al. (1986) both found that the PCT bore no relationship to any subsequent success in IVF. They concluded, though, that any couple with a negative PCT should consider IVF as a therapy for their infertility.

The other major test for sperm movement is the mucus penetration test (MPT), generally known as the Kremer test (Kremer 1965). This is a far better test than the PCT, as it allows controls to be developed as part of the test and can be carried out quite simply. In this test the migration of spermatozoa is tested in mucus from the male's partner and from a donor. No reports are available concerning the use of the MPT as a prognostic test for IVF but it does remain an important part of the work-up for any infertile couple. It enables some objective assessment of the capacity of the sperm to penetrate the cervical mucus and, if poor, may indicate the presence of either male or female sperm antibodies present or the presence of an "hostile mucus", i.e. a mucus which does not allow sperm penetration.

8.2.2.3 Sperm Capacitation

The capacitation of the sperm in vitro is important, for it has been shown, by observing the number of capacitated sperm at various time points, that the sperm in this situation capacitate at various times and in many cases there are spermatozoa which display delayed rates of capacitation (Reyes et al. 1984; Burkman 1984). As it has been shown that sperm which have not capacitated cannot penetrate zona-free hamster eggs (Rogers 1978), this suggests that insufficient numbers of capacitated sperm in vitro may lead to a reduced fertilization rate. Confirming this situation in a patient may explain a lack of fertilization and may also suggest sperm dysfunction.

The methods required to test the process of capacitation revolve around the ability to determine the presence of the sperm acrosome. This can be done by the method of Talbot and Chacon (1982) which allows discrimination between live and dead sperm, as well as sperm which have undergone capacitation. A factor which may be involved with the process of capacitation is the structural integrity of the acrosome. Jeulin et al. (1986) have described a group of men with poor fertilization rates in IVF who displayed abnormal acrosomal morphology, such as small or malformed acrosomes. It seems that the role of capacitation and acrosomal morphology in the assessment of the male will play major roles in the future.

8.2.2.4 Sperm Penetration Assay

The most popular test for sperm function is the zona-free hamster egg test (Yanagamachi et al. 1976), known generally as the sperm penetration assay (SPA). The methods for this test have been well documented elsewhere. The SPA is thought to evaluate the various physiological changes that must occur in the spermatozoon to achieve fertilization. The most obvious of these are capacitation and the acrosome reaction, which must occur for the spermatozoon to be capable of penetrating the oocyte. It is also a test of the spermatozoon's ability to fuse with the vitelline membrane of the oocyte and undergo gamete fusion (Rogers 1985). Although this seems to be a limited bioassay of sperm function, correlations have been established with the SPA and IVF (Wolf et al. 1983; Margalioth et al. 1986). There have been discussions on the problems associated with the occurrence of false results with the SPA, such as a patient's sperm failing to penetrate hamster oocytes (in which case the assay should be repeated on another semen sample) and then fertilizing human oocytes in vitro, suggesting that the SPA test cannot be used to exclude patients from an IVF programme (Cohen et al. 1982b; Evans 1986; Aitken 1986). The major reasons for the discrepancies are unknown but may involve such factors as capacitation and sperm–zona binding. Furthermore, Rogers and colleagues (1983) found an unacceptably high coefficient of variation in the SPA test when a group of men were tested five times over a period of twelve months. Attempts to improve the SPA test include the use of ionophore A23187 and prostaglandin E_2 (Aitken et al. 1984; Aitken and Kelly 1985). The results of these modifications look promising, but it must be emphasized that to be of any use, the assay must be very carefully performed and as long as there are significant numbers of patients who fail the SPA and yet are able to fertilize human oocytes in vitro, the SPA will not be the definitive test of fertility that it was once hoped to be.

This section demonstrates that there are a large variety of complex procedures which can be added to the basic semen analysis to test for various sperm parameters. It is still too early to determine which of these tests are the right ones to use, though it seems obvious that the major interest will be in the areas of sperm function and movement characteristics.

8.3 Separation of Motile Sperm

Originally it was thought that the mere addition of the semen sample would be sufficient to allow fertilization to occur in vitro but this was found not to be so due to the inhibitory effects of seminal plasma upon fertilization (Kanwar et al. 1979; Reddy et al. 1979). Furthermore, the presence of leucocytes associated with infection decreased the probability of fertilization (Reddy et al. 1979; Berger et al. 1982; Cohen et al. 1985a). Additionally, the culture medium would induce capacitation and the acrosome reaction (Rogers 1978), both of which are required for fertilization to occur.

8.3.1 "Swim-up" Procedure

The earliest method of separating motile from the non-motile sperm and cellular debris was a migration technique, known as the "swim-up" (Lopata et al. 1976) or "sperm-rise" procedure (Drevius 1971). This involved layering media directly upon a semen sample which was then left to incubate for 45–60 minutes, after which the uppermost 75% of the layered medium containing the motile spermatozoa is removed (Harris et al. 1981). Unfortunately, this technique may leave residual traces of seminal plasma, hence it is recommended that washing of the sample containing the motile sperm be carried out by dilution and centrifugation.

A variation of this procedure is a centrifugation–migration technique, whereby the semen sample is washed once or twice by the addition of medium to the semen sample followed by centrifugation (McDowell et al. 1985; Andolz et al. 1987). The sperm pellet obtained from this step is then resuspended in a small volume of medium (0.5 ml) and, as described previously, the fresh medium is layered upon the resuspended sperm pellet. After incubation for 45–60 minutes, the uppermost portion, containing the motile sperm, is removed. In cases of poor sperm motility, the semen sample may be divided into several aliquots and allowed to swim-up in several tubes to increase the recovery of motile sperm (Andolz et al. 1987). This technique, when used with a medium containing antibiotics, has been shown to remove the microbes from the semen sample, thus alleviating any chance of infecting the oocyte after insemination (Wong et al. 1986). This technique is good for increasing the motility and percentage of abnormal forms in normal semen samples but has a poor recovery rate of motile sperm in subnormal samples (McDowell et al. 1985).

A modification of the swim-up technique is the addition of Ficoll (Pharmacia, Sweden), a density medium, to the resuspended sperm pellet, thus creating a density gradient interface (Harrison 1976; Cummins and Breen 1984). This allows only actively motile sperm to pass across it. This technique has been used to recover a higher number of motile sperm. The migration–centrifugation techniques have been criticized since they add further centrifugation and washing steps which may be deleterious to the spermatozoa. However, when centrifugation of the sample is at low forces, i.e. 300–400 g, and the washing steps are kept to a minimum (yet enough to remove the seminal plasma) the swim-up technique has been found to be simple and effective for normal semen samples. Another variation of the swim-up technique has been to layer highly purified hyaluronic acid onto the semen sample (Wikland et al. 1987). This method results in a high percentage of motile sperm being recovered; this is thought to be due to the high viscosity of the hyaluronic acid selecting sperm of extremely good motility.

Another variation on the standard migration technique is the migration–gravity sedimentation technique (Tea et al. 1984). This, in essence, is similar to the basic swim-up technique except that instead of using a standard test tube, a specially constructed system with two built-in concentric tubes is used. The medium is placed in both the inner and outer tube and then semen is layered beneath the media in the outer tube by a syringe with a fine gauge needle. This system is then allowed to incubate for 3–6 hours during which time the progressively motile spermatozoa swim over the edge of the central tube and then sediment on the bottom of the central conical tube. The sample is then collected from the central tube by aspiration. This technique was shown to be useful for normal semen samples and also for cases of mid to low sperm motility.

8.3.2   Albumin Columns

The use of albumin columns is another method for selecting spermatozoa by their inherent motility (Koper et al. 1979; Ben-Nun et al. 1980; Singer et al. 1980; Binor et al. 1982; Urry et al. 1983). A small volume of the semen sample, roughly 0.5 ml (which is usually diluted with medium containing 10% serum 1:2 or 1:3), is placed upon a small column containing medium supplemented with 7.5% albumin or, alternatively, several discontinuous layers of densities can be used (Perrone and Testart 1985). This mixture is then incubated at 37°C. for 1–2 hours, after which the bottom 0.5 ml of the column is removed and washed by dilution with fresh medium and then centrifuged. The washed final sample will contain the progressively motile sperm. Usually, this technique involves the setting up of several columns to enable a good recovery of the motile sperm.

A modification of this technique involves the setting up of the columns using several 1 ml insulin syringes and then placing a washed semen sample on top of the albumin column within the syringes (Koper et al. 1979; Ben-Nun et al. 1980). The column is incubated for 1 hour and then the bottom level of albumin drained and then washed. Both of the above techniques were found to be useful for both normal and oligozoospermic patients.

8.3.3   Glass Wool Columns

The use of glass wool filtration has been proposed as a method for improving the quality of semen samples from both normal and patients with male infertility (Broer and Dauber 1977; Paulson and Polakoski 1977; Jeyendran et al. 1986). This method is based upon the filtering of a semen sample through a Pasteur pipette packed loosely with glass wool, after which there is an increase in the percentage of motile sperm and there is also a removal of debris and agglutinated and dead sperm (Paulson and Polakoski 1977). It has been reported that there may be some damage to the ultrastructure of spermatozoa passing through the glass wool column (Sherman et al. 1981) but testing of the spermatozoa after filtering by the HOS test has shown that the spermatozoa retain the integrity of their membranes (Jeyendran et al. 1986). This technique is not in common use, especially for IVF, but pregnancies have been reported following the artificial insemination of semen after the use of this technique.

8.3.4 Sedimentation

The use of a sedimentation technique was developed mainly in an attempt to improve sperm recovery for the treatment of male factor infertility in IVF (Cohen et al. 1984a,b. 1985a,b). The technique involves the washing of the semen sample by dilution with media and centrifugation. The sample is then resuspended in a small volume and divided into small aliquots (0.05–0.1 ml). The aliquots are placed on culture dishes and then covered with paraffin oil and stored in a 5% CO_2 atmosphere at either room temperature or at 4°C. The debris and non-motile sperm are allowed to settle out for 1–24 hours and then the top part of the droplet containing motile sperm is removed. In order to maximize sperm recovery by this technique, several samples were collected on every second day leading up to the time of insemination and stored. It was noted that in some cases a large portion of the motile sperm did fall into the sediment as well and that the presence of leucocytes negatively affected the number of motile sperm obtained in the final sample.

8.3.5 Percoll Gradients

In semen samples from patients with male factor infertility, the swim-up or the albumin column techniques often do not yield satisfactory results. This is due to there being poor motility in the original sample and, as these techniques rely upon the inherent motility of the sperm to separate themselves, poor separation often occurs. Percoll, a density gradient medium, has been used as a migration medium (Pousette et al. 1986), whereby motile sperm swim into Percoll gradient without any centrifugation. Its major use, however, has been as either continuous (Gorus and Pipeleers 1981; Arcidiacono et al. 1983) or discontinuous gradients with centrifugation (Forster et al. 1983; Dravland and Mortimer 1985; Hyne et al. 1986). The use of Percoll significantly decreases the amount of debris present, especially leucocytes (Gorus and Pipeleers 1981), and significantly increases the percentage of motile sperm (Berger et al. 1985).

With the use of discontinuous gradients, the isotonic Percoll is diluted with culture media to create solutions which are carefully layered upon each other in volumes of 1.5–2.0 ml. These solutions can vary in concentration from laboratory to laboratory, e.g. 40%, 55%, 70%, 80% and 90% (Berger et al. 1985); 40%, 60%, 70%, 80% (Kaneko et al. 1986). In a modification of the technique by Dravland and Mortimer (1985), just the use of a 45% and 90% gradients, in our hands, has been found to be quite successful. The gradient is then centrifuged at 200–300 g for 20–30 minutes. The higher concentrations of the Percoll gradient are removed (80% and greater), combined, diluted in culture medium, centrifuged and resuspended. Although this technique does, at first, seem relatively complex compared with the other techniques, it does become easier with practice and good results have been reported with the use of this technique, especially with samples from male factor infertility patients. Continuous gradients have also

been used (Bolton et al. 1984, 1986), although these require the use of a high
speed centrifuge to enable the self generation of the gradient.

The use of Percoll has also been shown to remove bacterial contamination
(Bolton et al. 1986) and has also been shown to select morphologically normal
forms of spermatozoa (Pousette et al. 1986). This may be important if, as some
studies suggest, the presence of high levels of abnormal forms may decrease the
rate of fertilization. There have been reports of there being some ultrastructural
damage to the spermatozoa (Arcidiacono et al. 1983), but as there have also been
reports of fertilization and pregnancy with the use of this material (Hyne et al.
1986), this does not seem to affect the fertilization process. Finally, in a
comparison of Percoll gradients, albumin columns and the swim-up technique as
methods of obtaining motile spermatozoa, the Percoll gradient was found to have
the highest percentage recovery of progressively motile sperm and also produced
a high percentage of motility in the final sample (Berger et al. 1985).

The question is therefore raised as to which is the best method to use. The swim-
up method is obviously the simplest method and, with normal semen samples, is
the obvious choice. However, once the problem of male factor infertility is
approached by an IVF clinic, the more specialized methods must come into play.
We have found that trial washes of the husband's semen sample, in cases of very
poor samples, has proved to be very helpful, as this allows any minor modifications to be made prior to the treatment cycle. Also, it allows several techniques to
be tried to assess which will be the best. In our experience, there is no one
technique which can be successfully used on every patient and several trials
may have to be made before the treatment cycle to establish a protocol for that
patient.

8.4   Male Factor Infertility

The studies of MacLeod and Gold (1951a,b,c) provided data concerning the
features of semen analyses from fertile and subfertile groups. These have been
subsequently revised in the light of additional large studies of men achieving
fertility, the tendency being to lower the lower limits of normality for sperm
concentration and motility (WHO 1987). Criteria accepted for normality in
studies sponsored by the WHO included sperm concentrations of greater than 20
$\times$ 10^6/ml, percentage motility greater than 50% and a percentage of normally
shaped sperm of 50% and greater (WHO 1987). However, there is an increasing
realization that men with semen parameters that are clearly below normal may
still achieve pregnancies. Analysis of such pregnancies indicate that even with
sperm concentrations of less than 5×10^6/ml, a cumulative pregnancy rate of 23%
can be achieved over the initial 2 years of infertility (Baker et al. 1986). Though
these rates are lower than those achieved in men with normal parameters, they
still represent a significant pregnancy rate which must be borne in mind in
designing studies of agents potentially influencing infertility or in determining the
time at which complex, expensive treatments, such as IVF, should be introduced
into their management.

In view of the basal pregnancy rate achieved by patients with lower than normal sperm concentrations with time, IVF should not be used early in the management of an infertile couple. For patients we included in a study of male factor infertility, there was a mean duration of infertility of 6 years and out of 150 patients, studied over a period of 3 years, there was a natural pregnancy rate of 3.5%, with 2.5% of the patients becoming pregnant prior to their IVF cycle and 1.5% of patients becoming pregnant after an IVF treatment cycle. Obviously, this is below the expected 5% pregnancy rate of male factor infertility.

8.4.1 IVF and Male Factor Infertility

With the discovery that relatively few spermatozoa were required for IVF, it was proposed that subnormal semen samples could be used to fertilize in vitro if sufficient numbers of spermatozoa could be obtained (Trounson 1982). Many IVF units have now used subnormal semen to achieve both fertilization and subsequent pregnancy.

Many IVF clinics have reported success with the treatment of male factor infertility but one of the major difficulties in comparing the data is that the selection criteria for male factor infertility patients varies. Table 8.1 provides a summary of some of the studies carried out in the area of male factor infertility. The presence of obvious aetiological factors in the female are recorded and the results of the subfertile men are grouped according to the presence or absence of such factors. In many cases, the description of the groups have been given as the semen parameters used for selection, rather than the generic name (i.e. oligozoospermia) for the definition of the various groups does vary from laboratory to laboratory. Any statistical differences that may have been recorded in the study have not been included, as this table is designed merely to give an overview and, as the statistical methods varied, this would make comparisons difficult. Case studies have not been included.

It can be seen that the use of subnormal semen samples compares well with that of normal samples and in most of the examples presented, even with a reduced fertilization rate, the pregnancy rate is as good as the overall results in the IVF clinic. Other studies into the use of subnormal semen in IVF have been carried out, such as that of Mahadevan and Trounson (1984). Also in another study the cumulus oophorus was removed from the oocyte with the use of hyaluronidase and also an attempt was made to stimulate the sperm (Mahadevan and Trounson 1985). In both of these cases, the number of male factor infertility patients was too small for conclusions to be made.

Cohen et al. (1984a,b, 1985a) report the successful use of IVF for male factor infertility. The patients classified as having male factor infertility were those with a sperm concentration of less than 10×10^6/ml and/or sperm motility less than 20% and/or abnormal morphology greater than 80%. There was found to be an overall fertilization rate of 57%, with the fertilization rate being 53% where only the male had an infertility factor and 59% where both couples had an infertility factor. There were cumulative pregnancy rates of 45% from 41 patients where the male alone was the contributing factor to the infertility and 26% where both partners had contributing factors. It must be noted that these are cumulative results, for many of the 41 patients had more than one treatment cycle. Unfortunately, the results per treatment cycle are not given.

Table 8.1. Studies on male factor and IVF

Study	Female factors	Male factors	Subgroups (no. of cycles)	%fert./ oocyte	%failed fert. cycle	%preg./ lapy	%preg./ transfer
Mahadevan et al., 1983	Patent tubes	Count <20 and/or motility	– (10)	15.6	N/A	N/A	N/A
	No patent tubes	<40 and/or abnormal morph. >40	– (13)	50.0	N/A	N/A	N/A
Mahadevan et al., 1985a	Both patent and non-patent	As above	– (63)	N/A	N/A	11	33
Battin et al., 1985		Count <10 and/or motility <30	Count <10 } 15	37.5	40	6.7[b]	11.1
			Motility <30	40.6	N/A	N/A	N/A
		+ positive SPA +	[a]Count >10	72.1	6.5	N/A	N/A
		abnormal morph. <40	[a]Motility >30	70.5	N/A	N/A	N/A
Naaktegboren et al., 1985	≥1 Patent tube	Count <15 and/or motility <50 and/or abnormal morph. >40	– (14)	13.0	27	8	33
			– (3)	39.0	N/A	N/A	N/A
Yovich et al., 1985	Various	Count <20	Motility <40 (9)	32.0	33	22[b]	33[b]
			Motility 40–60 (6)	50.0	17	17[b]	20[b]
			Motility >60 (4)	80.0	0	25[b]	25[b]
		Count >20	Motility <40 (27)	52.0	30	7	11
			Motility 40–60 (28)	86.0	0	7	7
			Motility >60 (82)[a]	77.0	5	12	13

[a] Not male factor group.
[b] Results calculated from data included in paper cited.
Count = sperm concentration $\times 10^6$/ml, motility = % motility, abnormal morphology = % spermatozoa with abnormal morphology, lapy = laparoscopy.

Jeulin et al. (1985) retrospectively divided male patients, regardless of sperm concentration, motility or morphology, into two groups on the basis of the cleavage of embryos after insemination. The discriminating factors between the group where there was successful embryo cleavage and the one with poor cleavage rates were parameters of sperm movement (specifically lateral head displacement) and sperm morphology (specifically the status of acrosomal morphology). These factors were especially pertinent after the washing and separating of the motile sperm, although they could be identified in the original sample.

It has been observed that, in male factor patients, suitable numbers of motile spermatozoa must be added to the oocyte for fertilization to occur. Van Uem et al. (1985) found that when a sperm concentration of less than 1.5×10^6/ml was used, no fertilization occurred. The patients in this study were described only as

Table 8.2. Results of study on male factor infertility and IVF

Study	Female factors	Male factors	Subgroups (no. of cycles)	%fert./ oocyte	%failed fert. cycle	%preg./ lapy	%preg./ transfer
This study	Various	Count <20 and/or motility	Motility <40 (18) (other values normal)	58.8	33	11	17
		<40 and/or abnormal morph. >60	[a]Motility 40–60 (24) (other values normal)	73.8	29	13	18
			Abnorm. morph. >60 (22) (other values normal)	78.0	14	18	21
			Count <5 (6) (other values normal)	59.3	17	0	0
			Count 5–20 (12) (other values normal)	64.9	17	12	20
			Motil. <40 & count >20 (17) (other values normal)	50.7	30	12	17
			Motil. <40 & ab. mor. >60 (14) (other values normal)	66.7	14	21	25
			Count <20 & ab. mor >60 (7) (other values normal)	60.9	14	29	33
			Motility <40, count <20 & abnormal morphology >60 (12)	6.4	75	0	0
		Antibodies	– (16)	46.3	44	25	44
			– (243)	67.0	11	16	18

[a] Normal.
Count = sperm concentration × 10^6/ml, motility = % motility, abnormal morphology = % spermatozoa with abnormal morphology, lapy = laparoscopy.

being oligozoospermic and no actual values were given as to what criteria were used to classify them. There was a 39.6% fertilization rate for this group of patients, compared to that of 88.6% for patients with normal semen parameters. There was a slightly lower pregnancy rate for couples with a male factor, although it is pointed out that the sample size of male factor patients used in the study was too small for any conclusions to be made.

Hirsch et al. (1986) classified males as having a male factor if the sperm concentration was less than 20×10^6/ml and/or sperm motility was less than 60% and/or greater than 40% abnormal forms and/or a score of less than two sperm penetrations in the SPA. Patients whose sperm displayed motility with poor forward progression were also classified as having a male factor. Although the fertilization rate was not given, there was a correlation found between low sperm concentrations and the fertilization rate, i.e. the lower the sperm concentration, the lower the fertilization rate. Overall, the SPA was found to have the best prognostic value in assessing the probability of fertilization. The pregnancy rate was higher than (or close to) that for couples where the male had normal semen parameters, although the values of the pregnancy rates are not given.

Hyne et al. (1986) carried out Percoll washes on low sperm concentration and motility male factor patients who had failed to fertilize in previous treatment cycles. The Percoll method used consisted of a discontinuous gradient, using three different concentrations. Using this method of preparation, there was a 34% fertilization rate. Although low, it must be remembered that this occurred in patients who had previously failed to fertilize any oocytes. There was a 60% pregnancy rate per treatment cycle but the sample size for this study was only five treatment cycles, so it is difficult to state whether Percoll specifically selects sperm that will maintain a high pregnancy rate. It does display that the Percoll wash does select sperm which are better capable of achieving fertilization.

The results from our ongoing study of male factor infertility are given in Table 8.2. All of the samples in this study were prepared by the centrifugation–migration technique. All of the results are given over the 32-month period in which the study has been carried out. It can be seen, in the majority of cases, that the fertilization rate compares extremely well with that of normal patients, as does the pregnancy rate. The group in which there was the greatest difficulty was where all the standard semen parameters were below normal (the triple defect group). The introduction of a Percoll wash has alleviated many problems with this group, increasing the fertilization rate to above 35%, and pregnancies have been established. Although the fertilization rate is reduced compared to the normal, this method displays an enormous increase when compared to the centrifugation–migration technique.

The use of IVF for male factor infertility is still a new area with the promise of newer techniques, such as microinjection and sperm stimulation, still on the horizon. The results from all groups indicate that IVF will be of major use in the future treatment of male factor infertility.

References

Aitken RJ (1986) Use of sperm–ova penetration tests to evaluate the infertile couple. In: Sauten RJ, Swerdloff RS (eds) Male reproductive dysfunction: diagnosis and management of hypogonadism, infertility and impotence. Marcel Dekker, New York, pp. 267–294

Aitken RJ, Kelly RW (1985) Analysis of the direct effects of prostaglandins on human sperm function. J Reprod Fertil 73:139–146

Aitken RJ, Best FSM, Richardson DW, Djahanbakhch O, Lees MM (1982) The correlates of fertilizing capacity in normal fertile men. Fertil Steril 38:68–76

Aitken RJ, Ross A, Hargreave T, Richardson D, Best FSM (1984) Analysis of human sperm function following exposure to the ionophore A23187. J Androl 5:321–329

Aitken RJ, Sutton M, Warner P, Richardson DW (1985) Relationship between the movement characteristics of human spermatozoa and their ability to penetrate cervical mucus and zona-free hamster oocytes. J Reprod Fertil 73:441–449

Amann RP, Hammerstedt RH (1980) Validation of a system for computerized measurements of spermatozoal velocity and percentage of motile sperm. Biol Reprod 23:647–656

Andolz P, Bielsa MA, Genesca A, Benet J, Egozcue J (1987) Improvement of sperm quality in abnormal semen samples using a modified swim-up procedure. Hum Reprod 2:99–101

Arcidiacono A, Walt H, Campana A, Balerna M (1983) The use of Percoll gradients for the preparation of subpopulations of human spermatozoa. Int J Androl 6:443–445

Atherton RW (1970) An objective method for evaluating Angus and Hereford sperm motility. Int J Fertil 20:109–112

Baker HW, Burger HG, de Kretser DM, Lording DW, McGowan P, Rennie GC (1981) Factors affecting the variability of semen analysis results in fertile men. Int J Androl 4:609–622

Baker HWG, Burger HG, de Kretser DM, Hudson B (1986) Relative incidence of etiological disorders in male infertility In: Santen RJ, Swerdloff RS (eds) Male reproductive dysfunction: diagnosis and management of hypogonadism, infertility and impotence. Marcel Dekker, New York, pp 341–372

Battin D, Vargyas JM, Sato F, Brown J, Marrs RP (1985) The correlation between in vitro fertilization of human oocytes and semen profile. Fertil Steril 44:835–838

Ben-Nun I, Lancet M, van der Van H, Scommegna A (1980) Separation of human spermatozoa from a single ejaculate into various age-groups. Int J Fertil 25:127–130

Berger RE, Karp LE, Williamson RA, Koehler J, Moore DE, Holmes LK (1982) The relationship of pyospermia and seminal fluid bacteriology to sperm function as reflected in the sperm penetration assay. Fertil Steril 37:557–564

Berger T, Marrs RP, Moyer DL (1985) Comparison of techniques for selection of motile spermatozoa. Fertil Steril 43:268–273

Binor Z, Rao R, van der Van H, Scommegna A (1982) The effect of albumin gradients and human serum on the longevity and fertilizing capacity of human spermatozoa in the hamster ova penetration assay. Fertil Steril 38:222–226

Bolton VN, Braude PR (1984) Preparation of human spermatozoa for in vitro fertilization by isopycnic centrifugation on self-generating density gradients. Arch Androl 13:167–176

Bolton VN, Warren RE, Braude PR (1986) Removal of bacterial contaminants from semen for in vitro fertilization or artificial insemination by the use of buoyant density centrifugation. Fertil Steril 46:1128–1132

Broer KH, Dauber U (1977) A filtering method for cleaning up spermatozoa in cases of asthenospermia. Int J Fertil 23:234–239

Burkman LJ (1984) Characterization of hyperactivated motility by human spermatozoa during capacitation: comparison of fertile and oligospermic sperm populations. Arch Androl 13:153–165

Clarke GN, Elliot PJ, Smaila C (1985) Detection of sperm antibodies in semen using the immunobead test: a survey of 813 consecutive patients. Am J Reprod Immunol Microbiol 7:118–123

Cohen J, Mooyart M, Vreeburg JTM, Yanagamachi R, Zeilmaker GH (1982a) Fertilizing ability and motility of spermatozoa from fertile and infertile men after exposure to heterologous seminal plasma. In Hafez ESE, Semm K (eds) Clinics in andrology: instrumental insemination. Martinus Nijhoff, The Hague, pp 53–78

Cohen J, Weber RFA, van der Vijver JCM, Zeilmaker GH (1982b) In vitro fertilizing capacity of human spermatozoa with the use of zona-free hamster ova: interassay variation and prognostic value. Fertil Steril 37:565–572

Cohen J, Fehilly CB, Fishel SB (1984a) Male infertility successfully treated by in vitro fertilization. Lancet I:1239

Cohen J, Edwards RG, Fehilly CB et al. (1984b) Treatment of male infertility by in vitro fertilization: factors affecting fertilization and pregnancy. Acta Euro Fertil 15:455–465

Cohen J, Edwards R, Fehilly C et al. (1985a) In vitro fertilization: a treatment for male infertility. Fertil Steril 43:422–432

Cohen J, Fehilly CB, Walters DE (1985b) Prolonged storage of human spermatozoa at room temperature or in a refrigerator. Fertil Steril 44:254–262

Cummins JM, Breen TM (1984) Separation of progressively motile spermatozoa from human semen by sperm rise through a density gradient. Aust J Med Lab 5:15–20

Dravland JE, Mortimer D (1985) A simple discontinuous Percoll gradient procedure for washing human spermatozoa. IRCS Med Sci 13:16–17

Drevius LO (1971) The "sperm-rise" test. J Reprod Fertil 24:427–429

Eliasson R (1971) Standards in evaluation of human semen. Andrologie 3:49–64

Evans JA (1986) Sperm penetration assay. Fertil Steril 45:141 (letter)

Forster MS, Smith WD, Lee WI, Berger RE, Karp LE, Stenchever, MA (1983) Selection of human spermatozoa according to their relative motility and their interaction with zona-free hamster eggs. Fertil Steril 40:655–660

Gorus FK, Pipeleers DG (1981) A rapid method for the fractionation of human spermatozoa according to their progressive motility. Fertil Steril 35:662–665

Harris SJ, Milligan MP, Masson GM, Dennis KJ (1981) Improved separation of motile sperm and its application to artificial insemination. Fertil Steril 36:219–221

Harrison RAP (1976) A highly efficient method for washing mammalian spermatozoa. J Reprod Fertil 48: 347–353

Hirsch I, Gibbons WE, Lipshultz L et al. (1986) In vitro fertilization in couples with male factor infertility. Fertil Steril 45:659–664

Holt WV, Moore HDM, Hillier SG (1985) Computer assisted measurement of sperm swimming speed in human semen: correlation of results with in vitro fertilization assays. Fertil Steril 44:112–119

Hyne RV, Stojanoff A, Clarke GN, Lopata A, Johnston WIH (1986) Pregnancy from in vitro fertilization of human eggs after separation of motile spermatozoa by density gradient centrifugation. Fertil Steril 45:93–96

Janick J, MacLeod J (1970) The measurement of human spermatozoal motility. Fertil Steril 21:140–146

Jenks JP, Cosentino MJ, Cockett ATK (1982) Evaluating sperm motility: a comparison of the Rochester motility scoring system versus videomicrography. Fertil Steril 38:756–759

Jeulin C, Feneux D, Serres C et al. (1986) Sperm factors related to failure of human in vitro fertilization. J Reprod Fertil 76:735–744

Jeyendran RS, Perez-Pelaez M, Crabo BG (1986) Concentration of viable spermatozoa for artificial insemination. Fertil Steril 45:132–134

Kamidono S, Hamaguchi T, Okada H, Hazama M, Matsumoto O, Ishigami J (1984) A new method for rapid spermatozoal concentration and motility: A multiple exposure photography system using the Polaroid camera. Fertil Steril 41:620–624

Kamidono S, Hazama M, Matsumoto O, Takada K, Tomioka O, Ishigamai J (1982) Study on human spermatozoal motility: Preliminary report on newly developed multiple exposure photography method Andrologia 15:111–119

Kaneko S, Oshio S, Kobanawa K, Kobayashi T, Mohri H, Iizuka R (1986) Purification of human sperm by a discontinuous Percoll density gradient with an intercolumn. Biol Reprod 35: 1059–1063

Kanwar KC, Yanagamachi R, Lopata A (1979) Effects of human seminal plasma on fertilizing capacity of human spermatozoa. Fertil Steril 31:321–327

Katz DF, Dott HM (1975) Methods of measuring swimming speed of spermatozoa, J Reprod Fertil 45:263–272

Katz DF, Overstreet JW (1981) Sperm motility assessment by videomicrography. Fertil Steril 35:188–193

Koper A, Evans PR, Witherow RO'N, Flynn JT, Bayliss M, Blandy JP (1979) A technique for selecting and concentrating the motile sperm from semen and oligospermia. Br J Urol 51:587–590

Kremer J (1965) A simple sperm penetration test. Fertil Steril 35:188–193

Liu YT, Warme PK (1977) Computerized evaluation of sperm cell motility. Comput Biomed Res 10:127–138

Lopata A, Patullo MJ, Chang A, James B (1976) A method for collecting motile spermatozoa from human semen. Fertil Steril 27:677–684

MacLeod J, Gold RZ (1951a) The male factor in fertility and infertility. II. Spermatozoon counts in 1000 men of known fertility and in 1000 cases of infertile marriage J Urol 66:436–449

MacLeod J, Gold RZ (1951b) The male factor in fertility and infertility. III. An analysis of motile activity in the spermatozoa of 1000 fertile men and 1000 men in infertile marriage. Fertil Steril 2:187–204

MacLeod J, Gold RZ (1951c) The male factor in fertility and infertility. IV. Sperm morphology in fertile and infertile marriage. Fertil Steril 2:394–414

Mahadevan MM, Trounson AO (1984) The influence of seminal characteristics on the success rate of human in vitro fertilization. Fertil Steril 42:400–405

Mahadevan MM, Trounson AO (1985) Removal of the cumulus oophorus from the human oocyte for in vitro fertilization. Fertil Steril 43:263–267

Mahadevan MM, Trounson AO, Leeton JF (1983) The relationship of tubal blockage infertility of an unknown cause, suspected male infertility and endometriosis to success of in vitro fertilization and embryo transfer. Fertil Steril 40:755–762

Mahadevan MM, Leeton JF, Trounson AO, Wood C (1985) Successful use of in vitro fertilization for patients with persisting low-quality semen. Ann NY Acad Sci 442:293–300

Makler A (1978) A new multiple exposure photography method for objective human spermatozoal motility determination. Fertil Steril 30:192–199

Makler A (1979) Simultaneous differentiation between motile, non-motile, live and dead human spermatozoa by combining supravital staining and multiple exposure photography procedures Int J Androl 2:32–42

Makler A (1980) Use of the elaborated multiple exposure photography (MEP) method in routine sperm motility analysis and for research purposes. Fertil Steril 33:160–166

Makler A, Itskovitz J, Brandes JM, Paldi E (1979) Sperm velocity and percentage of motility in 100 normospermic specimens analysed by the multiple exposure photography (MEP) method. Fertil Steril 31:155–161

Makler A, Tatcher M, Mohilever J (1980) Sperm semi-autoanalysis by a combination of multiple exposure photography (MEP) and computer techniques. Int J Fertil 25:62–66

Margalioth EJ, Navot D, Laufer N, Lewin A, Rabinowitz R, Schenker JG (1986) Correlation between the zona-free hamster egg sperm penetration assay and human in vitro fertilization. Fertil Steril 45:665–670

Matson PL, Tuvik AI, O'Halloran F, Yovich JL (1986) The value of the postcoital test in predicting the fertilization of human oocytes. J In Vitro Fertil Embryo Transfer 3:110–113

McDowell JS, Veeck LL, Jones, HW (1985) Analysis of human spermatozoa before and after processing for in vitro fertilization J In Vitro Fertil Embryo Transfer 2:23–26

Milligan MP, Harris S, Dennis, KJ (1980) Comparison of sperm velocity in fertile and infertile groups as measured by time-lapse photography. Fertil Steril 34:509–511

Mortimer D (1985) The male factor in infertility. I. Semen analysis. Curr Prob Obstet Gynaecol Fertil 8:1–87

Mortimer D (1986) A microcomputer-based semi-automated system for human sperm movement analysis. Clin Reprod Fertil 4:283–295

Naaktgeboren N, Devroey P, Traey E, Wisanto A, Van Steirteghem AC (1985) Success of in vitro fertilization and embryo transfer in relation to the causes of infertility. Acta Euro Fertil 16:281–287

Overstreet JW, Katz DF, Hanson FW, Fonseca JR (1979) A simple inexpensive method for objective assessment of human sperm movement characteristics. Fertil Steril 31:162–172

Paulson JD, Polakoski KL (1977) A glass wool column procedure for removing extraneous material from the human ejaculate. Fertil Steril 28:178–182

Perrone D, Testart J (1985) Use of bovine serum albumin column to improve sperm selection for human in vitro fertilization. Fertil Steril 44:839–841

Poland ML, Moghissi KS, Giblin PT, Ager JW, Olsen JM (1985) Variation of semen measures within normal men. Fertil Steril 44:396–400

Pousette A, Akerlof E, Rosenborg L, Fredricsson B (1986) Increase of progressive motility and improved morphology of human spermatozoa following their migration through Percoll gradients. Int J Androl 9:1–13

Reddy JM, Stark RA, Zaneveld LJD (1979) A higher molecular weight antifertility factor from human seminal plasma. J Reprod Fertil 57:437–446

Reyes A, Martinez R, Luna M, Chavarria ME, Merino G (1984) Quantitative evaluation of the human spermatozoal motility and acrosome reaction in infertile oligozoospermic and fertile euspermic men. Arch Androl 12:187–194

Rogers BJ (1978) Mammalian sperm capacitation, fertilization in vitro: a critique of methodology. Gamete Res 1:165–223

Rogers BJ (1985) The sperm penetration assay: its usefulness reevaluated. Fertil Steril 43:821–840

Rogers BJ, Perreault SD, Bentwood BJ, McCarville C, Hale RW, Soderdahl DW (1983) Variability in the human–hamster in vitro assay for fertility evaluation. Fertil Steril 39:204–211

Sherman JK, Paulson JD, Liu KC (1981) Effect of glass wool filtration on ultrastructure of human spermatozoa. Fertil Steril 36:643–647

Singer R, Sagiv M, Barnet M (1980) Properties of spermatozoa from normospermic and oligospermic human semen fractionated on columns of discontinuous gradients of albumin. Int J Fertil 25:51–56

Singer SL, Lambert H, Overstreet JW, Hanson FW, Yanagamachi R (1985) The kinetics of human sperm binding to the human zona pellucida and zona-free hamster oocyte in vitro. Gamete Res 12:29–39

Talbot P, Chacon RS (1981) A triple-stain technique for evaluating normal acrosomal reactions of human sperm. J Exp Zool 215:201–208

Tea NT, Jondet M, Scholler R (1984) A migration–gravity sedimentation method for collecting motile spermatozoa from human semen In: Harrison RF, Bonnar J, Thompson W (eds) Studies in fertility and sterility: in vitro fertilization, embryo transfer and early pregnancy. MTP Press, Lancaster, pp 13–18

Timouran H, Watchmaker G (1970) Determination of spermatozoan motility. Dev Biol 21:62–72
Tjoa WS, Smolensky MH, Hsi BP, Steinberger E, Smith KD (1982) Circannual rhythm in human
    sperm count revealed by serially independent sampling. Fertil Steril 38:454–459
Trounson AO (1982) Current perspectives of in vitro fertilization and embryo transfer. Clin Obstet
    Gynaecol 1:55–65
Urry RL, Middleton RG, McNamara L, Vikari CA (1983) The effect of single-density bovine serum
    albumin columns on sperm concentration, motility and morphology. Fertil Steril 40:666–669
Van Uem JFHM, Acosta AA, Swanson RJ et al. (1985) Male factor evaluation in in vitro fertilization:
    Norfolk experience. Fertil Steril 44:375–383
Wikland M, Wik O, Steen Y, Qvist K, Soderlund B, Janson PO (1987) A self-migration method for
    preparation of sperm for in vitro fertilization. Hum Reprod 2:191–195
Wolf DP, Sokoloski JE, Quigley MM (1983) Correlation of human in vitro fertilization with the
    hamster egg bioassay. Fertil Steril 40:53–59
Wong PC, Balmaceda JP, Blanco JD, Gibbs RS, Asch RH (1986) Sperm washing and swim-up
    technique using antibiotics removes microbes from human semen. 45:97–100
World Health Organization (1987) WHO laboratory manual for the examination of human semen and
    semen-cervical mucus interaction. Cambridge University Press, Cambridge
Yanagamachi R, Yanagamachi H, Rogers BJ (1976) The use of zona-free animal ova as a test system
    for the assessment of fertilizing capacity of human spermatozoa. Biol Reprod 15:471–476
Yovich JL, Stanger JD, Yovich JM (1985) The management of oligospermic infertility by in vitro
    fertilization. Ann NY Acad Sci 442:276–286
Zavos PM (1985a) Characteristics of human ejaculates collected via masturbation and a new Silastic
    seminal fluid collection device. Fertil Steril 43:491–492
Zavos PM (1985b) Seminal parameters of ejaculates collected from oligospermic and normospermic
    patients via masturbation and at intercourse with the use of a Silastic seminal fluid collection
    device. Fertil Steril 44:517–520

9 Oocyte Freezing

C. Chen

9.1 Introduction

The advent of in vitro fertilization (IVF) heralds a new era in our understanding and management of human infertility. It represents a major breakthrough in the field of human reproduction and affords hope for couples who desperately want a child of their own. Perhaps IVF can be regarded as one of the most important advances in reproductive medicine of this century.

Although IVF is now becoming widely practised in many parts of the world, its results are variable. In real terms the success rate world-wide has not shown any remarkable improvement over recent years; the average pregnancy rate per treatment cycle is in the order of 15%, with a "baby take-home rate" of less than 10% per course of treatment.

To obtain even these results, experience among established IVF programmes has clearly shown that the chances of achieving pregnancy in a single treatment cycle is very much dependent on the number of fertilized eggs replaced in utero. Thus the chance of pregnancy occurring if one embryo were implanted is 16%, and this chance is doubled with two, and better with three or more implanted (National Perinatal Statistics Unit 1985). There is therefore a need for obtaining a large number of oocytes in order to optimize the production of embryos for replacement. This has led to the use of a variety of ovarian stimulation regimens, employing various combinations of clomiphene citrate (CC), human menopausal gonadotrophin (hMG), and follicle stimulating hormone (FSH), in order to optimize the production of eggs.

Unfortunately such an approach carries with it the problem of a surplus production of eggs, and consequently of embryos which, if implanted in utero, increases the risk of multiple pregnancy. The occurrence of IVF twin, triplet and quadruplet pregnancies is well recognized (Chen et al. 1982; Kerin et al. 1983). The incidence in Australia alone of IVF twin pregnancy is 20%, and of triplets 3%, among all IVF pregnancies (National Perinatal Statistics Unit 1985). There is also the potential problem of serious disturbance to the hormonal support of the luteal phase, such as luteal phase defects, following the use of such stimulation regimens, thereby jeopardizing the chances of a successful implant (Garcia et al. 1981).

In order to minimize the risk of multiple pregnancy occurring, yet giving the patient a reasonable chance of success, many IVF programmes have adopted the approach of replacing regularly at embryo transfer no more than three or four embryos. Such a policy obviously creates a problem of surplus embryos, produced as a result of the fertilization of large numbers of oocytes obtained in any single treatment cycle. The excess embryos thus created will therefore require to be disposed of, a situation which raises a spectre of complex ethical, social, legal, moral and religious issues which will have to be confronted. A practical solution of this dilemma is to preserve the embryos through deep freezing. Unfortunately, cryopreservation serves only to postpone confrontation of the realities of these problems. Many religious groups are opposed to embryo cryopreservation because of their belief that the embryo is the beginning of human life. Therefore, subjecting embryos to cryopreservation would risk their destruction during the process of freeze–thawing as not all embryos will survive the process. Legal problems can also follow embryo cryopreservation. This was highlighted by the legal nightmare and controversy that followed the tragic death, through an aeroplane accident, of the parents of the Rios' frozen embryos (Hughes and McClusky 1984). These "orphaned" embryos suddenly became "unwanted" with their fate uncertain and, after much legal and moral debate, probably will be donated to another couple.

An alternative approach to the problem of spare or surplus embryos is to inseminate the required number of oocytes, and to store the excess oocytes by cryopreservation for later use, as and when the need arises. With the current controversy surrounding embryo freezing, there is clearly a need to explore the possibility of cryopreservation of the human oocyte as an alternative to embryo freezing in IVF programmes. Like sperm banking, oocyte storage should be more acceptable to the community, since the procedure involves only the gamete, and is therefore free of the encumberances associated with the storage of frozen human embryos. Of equal importance is the need for research into cryopreservation of the human oocyte. Little is known of the effects of deep freezing on the oocyte, its survival after thawing, and its subsequent performance and development following exposure to sperm in the IVF system. The potential significance and practical application of this research is clearly far-reaching.

9.2   The Human Oocyte

From the point of view of oocyte freezing, an important feature of the mammalian egg is its size. The oocyte at the time of ovulation is generally the largest cell found in most mammals, being a sphere varying in diameter from about 70–80 μm in the mouse to about 130 μm in the human. The oocyte is surrounded by a transparent non-cellular membrane, the zona pellucida, and a layer of follicular cells, the corona radiata. The ovum is therefore only just visible to the naked eye as a tiny white speck.

9.2.1 Oocyte Meiosis and Maturation

During intra-uterine life, as the ovary develops, oocytes enter the prophase of the first meiotic division, and then become arrested in the diplotene stage. This stage extends through infancy until just prior to the onset of puberty. With the onset of reproductive life, the meiotic process is resumed and the first meiotic division is then completed. The second meiotic division occurs and the oocyte is ovulated at the metaphase II stage, with the first polar body extruded, and the chromosomes arranged on a spindle at the second meiotic metaphase. Meiotic division then arrests again at this second phase. During this stage the oocyte may be regarded as relatively unstable. It is fairly characteristic of ovulated eggs that if fertilization does not occur, the spindle subsequently breaks down, the chromosomes forming micronuclei. It is the view of cryobiologists that the oocyte should best be cryopreserved at the ovulated phase (Polge 1977). Following fertilization, resumption of meiotic maturation occurs, and the second polar body is extruded.

9.3 Feasibility of Oocyte Cryopreservation

9.3.1 Animal Evidence

Attempts have been made in the past to preserve mammalian oocytes at very low temperatures. Early work in the 1950s provides evidence of this research although with little success. Thus Sherman and Lin (1958a,b, 1959) using unfertilized ovulated mouse oocytes and glycerol as cryoprotectant, obtained survival among oocytes when cooled to $-10\,°C$. None of them, however, survived below $-20\,°C$. The most significant demonstration in the 1950s of the survival of oocytes after freezing and thawing was provided by Parkes (1958) in experiments on slices of rat ovaries which after freeze–thawing were tested for viability by subcutaneous grafting. Although all the oocytes within graafian follicles appeared to be degenerating, numerous primordial follicles survived freezing. Parrott (1960) in a later study showed that mouse ovarian tissue when subjected to freeze–thawing at $-79\,°C$, and then grafted into the ovarian capsule of recipient mice, resulted in ovulation and healthy live births.

A temporary lull ensued until the 1970s when interest was again revived. Leibo (1977), in a study of mouse ova and embryos, obtained a higher proportion of ova surviving after deep freezing to $-196\,°C$. Survival was found to bear an inverse relationship to cooling rates and the formation of intracellular ice. These observations were fundamental to an understanding of the cryobiological processes involving cells held at very low temperatures. In another equally important study, Whittingham (1977), using dimethyl sulphoxide (DMSO) as cryoprotectant, succeeded not only in cooling unfertilized ovulated mouse oocytes to a temperature of $-196\,°C$, permitting storage from between 24 hours to 3 months, but also obtained 70% survival among those oocytes, thus clearly demonstrating the feasibility of oocyte cryopreservation. Fertilization in vitro of the frozen–thawed oocytes was significantly lower than those of freshly collected control oocytes. However, live healthy normal fetuses were obtained after transfer of the oocytes into the oviducts of recipient females when mated with fertile males. Successful oocyte cryopreservation was later achieved by Kasai et al. (1979) in the rat. The oocytes were frozen at −196 °C using DMSO, with 60% surviving after thawing and 47% demonstrating fertilization in vitro.

Parkening and Chang (1977) have stored hamster oocytes at −75 °C, whilst Quinn et al. (1982) obtained an 80% survival of these oocytes after slow cooling to −80 °C prior to storage at −196 °C. All the ova in Quinn's study were penetrated by mouse spermatozoa, indicating that the freezing procedure did not adversely affect hamster ova penetration by heterologous spermatozoa. In a more recent study by De Mayo et al. (1985), an attempt was made to freeze monkey oocytes as a forerunner to similar procedures in the human. The monkey oocytes were collected by laparoscopy after appropriate ovarian hyperstimulation, and then frozen in DMSO before storage at −196 °C. Ova were stored for between 1 and 12 weeks in liquid nitrogen. The stored ova were thawed either slowly or rapidly and then subjected to xenogenous fertilization in the rabbit oviduct. Survival after freeze–thawing varied between 20% to 40%, with xenogenous fertilization rates of around 30%.

9.3.2 Human Studies

Whilst animal studies clearly showed that the mammalian oocyte could be successfully frozen and stored, there was little evidence to indicate that this could be possible in man. Indeed, it was thought by some IVF researchers that cryopreservation of the human oocyte was extremely difficult, if not technically impossible, because of the potential instability of the oocyte chromosome spindle when subjected to freezing and thawing. In one study, however, 10 human ova were exposed to 35% glycerol and then frozen in liquid nitrogen (Burks et al. 1965). Nine retained their morphological integrity after thawing. In another study, Trounson (1984) obtained more than 80 oocytes from ovarian wedge samples and cultured them for 48 hours in vitro prior to freezing. Only four oocytes survived both freezing and subsequent thawing. In yet another study, Bernard et al. (1985), using glycerol as cryoprotectant, found that none of their oocytes were fertilizable after freeze–thawing. In the same study in which 1,2-propanediol was used instead, both fertilization and cleavage to the 8-cell stage occurred in one egg before the experiment was terminated. There was, however, insufficient description of details of the actual freeze–thaw processes involved.

9.4 Cryobiological Concepts in Oocyte Cryopreservation

9.4.1 Cryobiological Concepts

Before undertaking work on oocyte cryopreservation, an understanding of cryobiological concepts in cell freezing is an essential prerequisite. Successful freeze-preservation is attributable to the application of theoretical considerations and empirical observations derived from studies in other species and cellular systems. There are, indeed, two factors of utmost importance in cryopreservation work: the presence of molar concentration of a protective solute or cryoprotectant, and appropriate rates of cooling and warming. Cryoprotective solutes which are of low molecular weight are thought to prevent the potentially deleterious exposure of cells to elevated concentrations of electrolytes by their colligative action in reducing the quantity of ice formed intracellularly at any sub-zero temperature. Also, precise control of the cooling rate and warming rate determines the ultimate fate of water present intracellularly during the cryopreservation process.

If during freezing the rate of cooling is sufficiently slow, cytoplasmic water will flow out of the cell and freeze extracellularly, resulting in a gradual dehydration of the cell. However, damage to the cell at slow rates of cooling may be caused by solution effects, which in turn can be reduced by the use of cryoprotective media. On the other hand, if cooling is too rapid, the cytoplasm will not have sufficient time to dehydrate, it will supercool, and eventually freeze. The formation of intracellular ice is thought to lead to cell damage and death. For different cells there is an optimal cooling rate which varies according to the cell type.

9.4.2 Cellular Events During Freezing and Thawing

When a cell suspended in a physiological medium is cooled progressively to temperatures slightly below 0 °C, ice forms first in the extracellular solution. Consequently, the dissolved solutes become more concentrated as water is removed in the form of ice. As the temperature of the cell suspension is lowered further, more ice forms, resulting in a progressively more concentrated extracellular solution. The higher the concentration, the lower the chemical potential of water. The cell responds osmotically to equalize the chemical potentials of water across its membranes; hence during freezing, it loses water extracellularly. If the cell is cooled sufficiently slowly, it will progressively lose more water as the temperature is lowered so as to maintain an osmotic equilibrium with the extracellular solution. However, if a cell is cooled at high enough rates, there will be insufficient time for the cell to remain in osmotic equilibrium and, as the temperature falls, the cell contents will become increasingly supercooled, until suddenly the cell water freezes within the cell itself, thereby resulting in cell death. Seeding, or the induction of ice formation in the medium, overcomes this problem of supercooling and the deleterious effect of thermal changes following the release of the latent heat of fusion.

As cooling proceeds further, and the temperature reaches −40 °C, 74% of the solution becomes crystallized and the solute concentration in the remaining liquid increases to 47 weight % (Rall et al. 1984). Many small ice crystals form and surround the cell, thereby obscuring it from view on cryomicroscopy. The next phase is a critical one where cell death can occur. As the temperature falls further, the intracellular contents freeze and the cell suddenly reappears. This is caused by the diffraction of light by the ice crystals formed intracellularly – a phenomenon termed "blackening out" or "flashing". If the cell is now cooled rapidly by plunging it into liquid nitrogen at −196 °C, there is no additional crystallization, that is, a "glass" forms and the residual liquid "vitrifies". Cooling to −196 °C results in an arrest of biological time for the cell, which can then be stored virtually indefinitely.

On thawing, the physical events depend on whether warming is slow or rapid. Slow warming is accompanied by a complex series of changes: a "flashing" of the cytoplasm at -90 °C, "first flash", the gradual growth of a dark crystalline material extracellularly between -90 °C to -70 °C, gradual disappearance of the dark material between -70 °C to -42 °C, and a "second flash" at -55 °C. With rapid warming, that is, rates in excess of 100 °C/minute, the extracellular ice merely melts when the temperature increases above -40 °C. There is insufficient time for the formation of ice nuclei or "devitrification" and the glassy solid therefore "liquefies". The final step is a critical one of diluting out the cryoprotectant and a return to physiological conditions.

These cryobiological concepts described are clearly of great importance. The role of the cryoprotectant in protecting the cell during freezing, the avoidance of supercooling by seeding, careful control of the rate of cooling, the prevention of significant intracellular ice formation, the establishment of osmotic and thermal equilibrium during freezing, and the control of warming rates are of paramount concern. Both an understanding of these concepts, and meticulous attention to and control of these factors during freezing and thawing, are influential in a successful outcome of the cryopreservation process.

9.5   Developing Oocyte Freezing Using an Animal Model

In order to establish oocyte cryopreservation at the Flinders Medical Centre in Adelaide, a murine model was used initially to develop the technique of freezing (Chen 1986). Three- to 4-week-old female mice belonging to an F_1 hybrid strain derived by crossing C57BL with CBA were superovulated using a combination of pregnant mare's serum gonadotrophin 10 IU and human chorionic gonadotrophin (hCG) 10 IU given 48 hours later. Both ovulated and fertilized oocytes were harvested on the morning after hCG administration and used for freezing.

Various factors which were thought to influence successful cryopreservation were investigated, and included the volume of Dulbecco's phosphate buffered saline (PBS) for suspending the oocytes during freezing, the concentration of DMSO as cryoprotectant, the method of seeding, the temperature at which seeding was induced, the rate of freezing, the rate of thawing, and the final removal of DMSO prior to culture in vitro. Oocyte survival was assessed morphologically, and signs of damage such as zonal disruption, discoloration of the ooplasm, as well as pyknosis, observed. Survival of both ovulated and fertilized oocytes was observed morphologically. Further development of the fertilized oocytes was assessed by their continued development in culture in the laboratory.

The optimal volume of PBS required for suspending the oocyte during freezing was found to vary between 0.2 ml and 0.3 ml. Volumes in excess of this failed to freeze quickly at the seeding temperature. Seeding induced at temperatures above -5 °C was unsatisfactory, whereas at -7 °C freezing of the buffer was both rapid and efficient. The concentration of DMSO that gave optimal survival was 1.5 M, whilst the rate of freezing for the oocyte between the seeding and storage temperatures was 0.5 °C/minute. Experiments with the mouse oocyte also

Table 9.1. Survival of animal oocytes using the slow-freeze and fast-thaw technique

Reference	Species	Number	Survival (%)
Chen (1986)	Mouse	250	75
Pellicer et al. (1987)	Rat	79	67
Fugger (1987)[a]	Mouse	18	78

[a] Personal communication.

revealed that slow freezing should cease by $-40\,°C$, and the oocyte should then be rapidly frozen to $-196\,°C$ by immersion in liquid nitrogen before storage. Thawing had to be rapid as well, with rates exceeding $300\,°C$/minute, in order to optimize oocyte survival. This was obtained by immersion in a hot water-bath. Both the addition and removal of DMSO from the cell was achieved in a single or stepwise fashion. The morphological survival rates obtained by both the author and others using this slow-freeze and fast-thaw technique are shown in Table 9.1.

9.6 Establishing Human Oocyte Freezing

Having determined the optimal conditions for oocyte cryopreservation from the murine model, work then commenced on the human oocyte. A programme of IVF and embryo transfer (ET) established at the Flinders Medical Centre provided material for the study. Patients were being treated in the programme for a variety of indications. The majority, 81%, had a significant tubal factor as a cause for their infertility, whilst endometriosis, male factors and idiopathic infertility accounted for the remaining 19%.

The women were stimulated with CC given either alone or with hMG to achieve follicular development. A typical regimen involved the use of CC 100 mg given daily for 5 days from day 4 of the cycle, together with hMG 150 IU or more also given daily from day 6, until a satisfactory serum estradiol response was obtained. The pattern of this response, together with ultrasound evidence of follicular growth, was used to time the administration of hCG 5000 IU. Oocyte retrieval was performed by laparoscopy about 34 hours after the administration of hCG. When an endogenous surge of luteinizing hormone (LH) occurred, as revealed in either serum or 3-hourly urine samples, then retrieval was performed 26 hours from the time of the urinary surge.

The oocytes obtained were incubated at $37\,°C$ in a medium modified from Whittingham's formula. The medium used for fertilization and cleavage was supplemented with human serum, whilst the gas phase used during culture consisted of a special mixture of 5% carbon dioxide and oxygen, and 90% nitrogen. Insemination of the oocyte was usually delayed over several hours in order to permit oocyte maturation in vitro. Fertilization was usually assessed between 12 and 18 hours after insemination, at which time the medium was changed to one of higher serum concentration. Embryos were regularly transferred back to the patient at between the 2- and 6-cell stages, with the procedure being performed in the dorsal position, under mild sedation. No more than four embryos were replaced at any time, with the use of a simple Teflon catheter within a soft outer sleeve. Post-transfer monitoring included serial serum progesterone assays and, when indicated, the measurement of β-hCG by radioimmunoassay. Oocytes in excess of those required to establish four embryos were then used for freezing after culture for varying periods of time in order to allow further maturation in vitro.

9.7   Factors Influencing Successful Freezing

A systematic study was made of various factors which were thought to affect the successful outcome of human oocyte freezing and thawing. They included oocyte quality and maturation, the size of the oocyte–cumulus oophorus complex, the volume of freezing medium, the use of cryoprotectant, the seeding technique, and the rate of freezing and thawing.

9.7.1   Criteria for Oocyte Selection

Not all oocytes were found suitable for freezing. Those that appeared morphologically normal, with a well-dispersed cumulus, and where the hormonal profiles during ovarian stimulation in the treatment cycle looked good, seemed to perform well.

9.7.2   Stage of Oocyte Maturation

The stage at which the maturing oocyte should be frozen was investigated. Before freezing, oocytes were cultured in vitro for several hours after their retrieval, in order to allow their maturation in vitro. The optimal interval between hCG administration or LH surge, and the commencement of freezing was determined. Both survival and fertilization with subsequent cleavage were observed most frequently 38–42 hours after hCG or an LH surge, by which time the oocyte should have matured to metaphase II.

9.7.3   Size of Oocyte–Cumulus Oophorus Complex

The size of the oocyte–cumulus complex as a factor influencing successful freezing was also investigated, since some reports have suggested that cell size could adversely affect freezing (Polge 1977). The size of the cumulus was reduced by brief exposure to pooled sperm-free human seminal plasma. Later, it was found that the same objective could be achieved using a mechanical rather than a chemical approach, by needle dissection. The oocyte was then washed twice in PBS which was supplemented with bovine serum albumin (from the Commonwealth Serum Laboratories, Melbourne, Australia) and 10% fetal bovine serum (from Flow Laboratories, NSW, Australia).

9.7.4 Volume of Medium for Freezing

The optimal volume of the medium to be used for suspending the oocyte during freezing was determined. Oocytes were frozen in a 1.2 ml cryule (from Wheaton Scientific, New Jersey, USA). A volume of 0.3 ml was found most satisfactory, permitting seeding to be completed rapidly and efficiently. Volumes exceeding this froze too slowly after seeding, and gave unsatisfactory results.

9.7.5 Exposure to DMSO

Although the addition of cryoprotectant as a one-step procedure was found to give acceptable results, the rapid stepwise addition of pre-chilled DMSO was preferred. The optimal final concentration of DMSO in the suspending medium within the cryule was 1.5 M. After transfer of the oocyte into a cryule, the oocyte was then equilibrated at 0 °C within an automatic cell freezer (Model R204, from Planer Products Ltd, UK) for 20 minutes.

9.7.6 Seeding

The temperature was later rapidly decreased to −7 °C, at which point seeding of the sample was induced by touching the outside of the ampoule at the level of the meniscus with cold forceps until the sample froze "solid". Seeding occurred best at −7 °C. A period of 20 minutes was allowed before proceeding with further cooling of the oocyte.

9.7.7 Rate of Freezing

The rate of cooling was 0.5 °C/minute between −36 °C and −40 °C; the oocyte was then rapidly cooled to −196 °C by immersion in liquid nitrogen, prior to storage. Again, this cooling rate was found to be favourable for the human oocyte. Cessation of slow cooling below −40 °C seemed to result in poor survival. Cooling rates that were too rapid also resulted in cell death.

9.7.8 Rate of Thawing

Thawing of the oocyte was performed rapidly at rates exceeding 500 °C/minute by immersion of the ampoule in a 45 °C water-bath. Slower rates of warming were found to be detrimental to the oocyte. The cryoprotectant was removed as a stepwise procedure, by the addition of four times the sample volume with PBS, and the oocyte then examined for morphological evidence of survival.

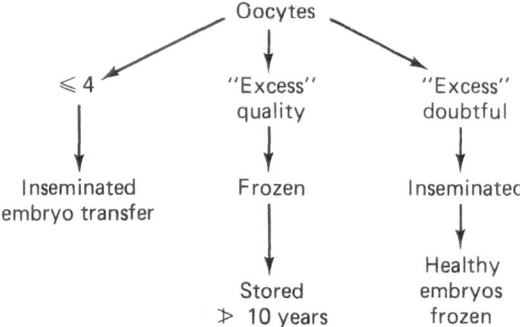

Fig. 9.1. Protocol for human oocyte cryopreservation.

9.7.9 Assessment of the Oocyte

The oocyte was observed for signs of cryodamage which included zonal fracture, discoloration of the ooplasm, cell disruption and pyknosis. Further assessment of the oocyte was obtained by transfer into the regular culture medium, and at the appropriate time, insemination performed with approximately 10 000 sperms/ml. The subsequent performance of the oocyte was observed by the appearance of fertilization and cleavage.

A suggested protocol for oocyte cryopreservation is shown in Fig. 9.1. Up to three or four oocytes may be used in regular IVF. Oocytes which appear to be of good quality, and are in excess of the three or four required for regular IVF may be frozen. Storage of these oocytes should not exceed 10 years. Oocytes which are of doubtful quality should not be used for freezing but should be inseminated and their performance judged before being considered for freezing as embryos.

9.8   Results of Human Oocyte Cryopreservation

The results obtained in an initial study of 40 human oocytes using the slow-freeze and rapid-thaw technique are given in Table 9.2 (Chen 1986). At least 80% of the

Table 9.2. Human oocyte survival after cryopreservation and its performance following insemination

Stage	Number of oocytes
Frozen	40
Survived	32 (80%)
Inseminated	30
Fertilized	25 (83%)
Cleaved	18 (60%)

From Chen (1986).

oocytes survived freezing and became fertilized on exposure to sperm, with 60% proceeding to cleavage division of 6- to 8-cell stages. Both the time of appearance of the pronuclei and cleavage rates were nearly similar compared with those of unfrozen fertilized oocytes.

9.8.1 Clinical Studies

Embryo transfers of two or three embryos derived from frozen–thawed oocytes were performed and two pregnancies resulted from seven patients treated.

The first patient to conceive was aged 29 with primary infertility of 7 years' duration, due to severe pelvic inflammatory disease which left her with bilateral hydrosalpinges. She had failed to conceive despite pelvic microsurgery and the performance of salpingostomies. She then underwent an IVF treatment cycle, following her last menstrual period on 9 October 1985, and received CC 100 mg daily with hMG. Her serum oestradiol peaked on day 11 with a mean follicular diameter of 19 mm on ultrasonography. Human chorionic gonadotrophin was given on cycle day 12, followed by a laparoscopy on day 14, which led to the recovery of six oocytes which were cryopreserved. Three of the oocytes were thawed subsequently and after a further 4 hours of culture, inseminated with 20 000 sperms/ml. The three frozen–thawed oocytes became fertilized, and were replaced in utero on day 16 at the 3- and 4-cell stages. She was advised to abstain from intercourse until the outcome of the transfer was known.

A β-hCG test gave a positive result by day 27 of her cycle. Subsequent serial assays showed normal results, with a level of 39 000 IU/ml on day 49. A healthy twin gestation was confirmed by ultrasonography at 7 weeks of gestation. The pregnancy progressed uneventfully and she was delivered of a healthy, normal set of twins on 4 July 1986 by elective Caesarean section at 38 weeks' gestation. The boy weighed 6 lb 4 oz, and the girl, 6 lb 5 oz. Chromosomal studies of their cord blood leucocyte cultures showed a normal male and female karyotype respectively, with banding studies confirming the results. Both children are developing normally.

Another woman to conceive with the same technique was aged 37 years, with primary infertility of 3 years because of bilateral tubal obstruction that remained despite tubal surgery. She had had IVF treatment since 1984 but failed to conceive after four attempts in spite of embryo implants in three. On the fourth attempt she received a total dose of CC 500 mg, hMG 900 IU and hCG 5000 IU. This resulted in the recovery of nine oocytes at laparoscopy, four of which became fertilized and were implanted but failed to produce a pregnancy; two failed to fertilize, and the remaining three were frozen and stored.

Four months later she returned for the replacement of her stored eggs during a natural cycle. An LH urinary surge was first detected on day 15, and the three oocytes were thawed 36 hours later. Two of the oocytes survived and were subsequently inseminated. They both fertilized and were implanted on day 18 at the 2- to 3-cell stages. Beta-hCG was detected on day 29 and the level of hCG continued to increase steadily. An ultrasound examination at 8 weeks' gestation confirmed the presence of a developing singleton pregnancy and amniocentesis revealed a normal female karyotype, with banding studies confirming the results. The pregnancy proceeded uneventfully to term with the birth of a normal female infant by Caesarean section. This baby is also developing normally.

9.9   Discussion

Contrary to the views expressed by other workers on the feasibility of cryopreservation of the human oocyte, this study clearly demonstrates that the pre-ovulatory oocyte can be successfully frozen and stored. Mammalian eggs had already been successfully cryopreserved at least 8 years previously by Whittingham (1977) who, in a classic study of mouse oocytes, clearly showed that ovulated oocytes could survive deep freezing at $-196\,^{\circ}C$ with a survival rate of around 70%. The mouse oocytes in his study were capable of fertilization in vitro, although with lower rates than control unfrozen oocytes, and on transfer to recipient females resulted in normal live-births. A slow-freeze and fast-thaw technique was used, which gave optimal rates of survival for both oocytes and embryos at various peri-implantation stages. However, the technique may not be applicable to the human oocyte, presumably because of species differences. It is recognized that there are structural differences between the chromosomes of mouse and man.

Parthenogenetic activation of the frozen–thawed human oocyte was not seen in the author's study, nor was the phenomenon observed among frozen mouse oocytes by Whittingham in his study. With the human oocytes there was clear morphological evidence of the appearance of both male and female pronuclei with subsequent syngamy and cell cleavage. At present the only practical means of assessing the survival and subsequent performance of the fertilized frozen–thawed human oocyte is by its morphological appearance on light microscopy. The application of chromosomal analysis and of electron microscopy for the investigation of the oocyte are areas for future study.

The risk of fetal malformation resulting from freeze–thawing of the human egg is not known. The findings of a normal karyotype among both frozen egg twins and the second pregnancy are both encouraging and reassuring. The studies of other species in which freeze–thawing has been effective have also shown no increased risk of fetal malformation. It is probable that only the more robust cells survive, and malformation may therefore be uncommon; certainly there is no evidence of an increased risk of malformation in mammalian or human embryos after freeze–thawing.

9.9.1   Practical Applications of Human Oocyte Cryopreservation

Although at a preliminary stage, the establishment of this method of human oocyte cryopreservation may have important implications. It may provide the prospect for storing surplus oocytes for use, when necessary, in subsequent unstimulated IVF cycles. The possibility also exists for the future establishment of oocyte banking. Thus women who suffer from diseases that endanger the life of the ovaries (such as cancer, endometriosis, recurrent cysts and infection) may wish to have their oocytes stored for future use. Should their ovaries require removal to cure the disease, they could still become pregnant through IVF, using their stored oocytes.

Oocyte freezing may provide a means for family planning. Thus, women who defer childbearing because of the pursuit of a career, the unavailability of a marriage partner, or ill health may at a young age opt to have their oocytes stored for later use. The storage of oocytes at the time of sterilization may also be of importance for those women who later regret the operation and desire a family, especially if a reversal operation should prove unsuccessful.

Stored oocytes may find their use in oocyte donation programmes to provide embryos for women with congenital or surgical absence of the ovaries, the presence of hypoplastic ovaries, the failure to produce ovulation from stimulation regimens, premature menopause, genetic diseases, and ovaries which are inaccessible to both laparoscopic and ultrasonic collection of oocytes.

9.9.2 Advantages of Human Oocyte Cryopreservation

As regimens for stimulating the production of more than one oocyte improve, it is commonplace for three or more oocytes to be collected in any treatment cycle. If more than three oocytes are obtained, then the excess numbers can be frozen and used to attempt conception at a later date. This has the advantages of a reduction in the risk of multiple pregnancy, the number of anaesthetics and laparoscopies a woman needs to undergo to achieve a pregnancy, a greater chance of success from embryo implants in a natural cycle, and a significant reduction in costs to the patient.

Oocyte freezing is also expected to increase the efficiency of IVF, by increasing the number of pregnancies from several eggs obtained in any single IVF treatment cycle. It also increases the patient's pregnancy potential, since several eggs obtained can be used in several future cycles. It may provide an alternative to embryo freezing. Oocyte cryopreservation should ultimately assist in alleviating some of the serious objections and concerns related to human embryo storage, and is expected to become more acceptable to the community.

9.9.3 Frozen Human Oocyte Pregnancies World-wide

To date, a total of five pregnancies derived from frozen human oocytes have been reported (Table 9.3). All have been achieved using a slow-freeze and fast-thaw technique, with DMSO as cryoprotectant. Three of the pregnancies have delivered; and all the infants, a male and three females, are healthy and normal. The remaining two pregnancies resulted in first trimester miscarriages. Although the development of the technique of human oocyte cryopreservation is difficult and is still in its infancy, the results obtained are encouraging and, in time, human oocyte cryopreservation should become an established procedure.

Table 9.3. Frozen human oocyte pregnancies reported

Reference		Pregnancies
Chen	1986	Twins (M+F)[a] delivered
(Adelaide, Australia)	1987	Single (F) delivered
van Uem et al.	1987	Single (F) delivered
(Erlangen, West Germany)		
Diedrich	1987	Miscarriages (2)
(Bonn, West Germany)		

[a] M, male; F, female.

References

Bernard A, Imoedemhe DA, Shaw RW, Fuller B (1985) Effects of cryoprotectants on human oocyte. Lancet I:632–633

Burks JL, Davis ME, Bakken AH, Tomasovic JJ (1965) Morphologic evaluation of frozen rabbit and human ova. Fertil Steril 16:638–641

Chen C (1986) Pregnancy after human oocyte cryopreservation. Lancet I:884–886

Chen C, Jones WR, Mudge TJ (1982) The development of an in vitro fertilization programme within an infertility service. Clin Reprod Fertil 1:327–330

De Mayo FJ, Rawlins RG, Dukelow WR (1985) Xenogenous and in vitro fertilization of frozen/ thawed primate oocytes and blastomere separation of embryos. Fertil Steril 43:295–300

Diedrich K (1987) Cryopreservation of rabbit and human oocytes. In: Abstracts of 5th world congress on in vitro fertilization and embryo transfer. Norfolk, Virginia, 5–10 April

Garcia J, Jones GS, Acosta A, Wright GL (1981) Corpus luteum function after follicle aspiration for oocyte retrieval. Fertil Steril 36:565–572

Hughes G, McClusky L (1984) $m embryos riddle. The Sun (Melbourne), 18 June

Kasai M, Iritani A, Chang MC (1979) Fertilization in vitro of rat ovarian oocytes after freezing and thawing. Biol Reprod 21:839–844

Kerin JF, Quinn PJ, Kirby C et al. (1983) Incidence of multiple pregnancy after in vitro fertilization and embryo transfer. Lancet II:537–540

Leibo SP (1977) Fundamental cryobiology of mouse ova and embryos. In: Elliot K, Whelan J (eds) The freezing of mammalian embryos. Elsevier Excerpta Medica, Amsterdam, pp 69–96 (Ciba Foundation 52 (new series))

National Perinatal Statistics Unit (1985) In vitro fertilization pregnancies, Australia and New Zealand, 1979–1984. National Perinatal Statistics Unit, Sydney

Parkening TA, Chang MC (1977) Effects of cooling rates and maturity of the animal on the recovery and fertilization of frozen–thawed rodent eggs. Biol Reprod 17:527–531

Parkes AS (1958) Factors affecting the viability of frozen ovarian tissue. J Endocrinol 17:337–343

Parrott DMV (1960) The fertility of mice with orthotopic ovarian grafts derived from frozen tissue. J Reprod Fertil 1:230–241

Pellicer A, Lightman A, De Cherney AH (1987) The importance of corona–cumulus complex to the survival and in vitro maturation of frozen–thawed rat oocytes. In: Abstracts of 5th world congress on in vitro fertilization and embryo transfer. Norfolk, Virginia, 5–10 April

Polge C (1977) The freezing of mammalian embryos: perspectives and possibilities. In: Elliott K, Whelan J (eds) The freezing of mammalian embryos. Elsevier Excerpta Medica, Amsterdam (Ciba Foundation 52 (new series)) pp 3–18

Quinn P, Barros C, Whittingham DG (1982) Preservation of hamster oocytes to assay the fertilizing capacity of human spermatozoa. J Reprod Fertil 66:161–168

Rall WF, Reid DS, Polge C (1984) Analysis of slow-warming injury of mouse embryos by cryomicroscopical and physicochemical methods. Cryobiology 21:106–121

Sherman JK, Lin TP (1958a) Survival of unfertilized mouse eggs during freezing and thawing. Proc Soc Biol Med 98:902–905

Sherman JK, Lin TP (1958b) Effect of glycerol and low temperature on survival of unfertilized mouse eggs. Nature 181:785–786

Sherman JK, Lin TP (1959) Temperature shock and cold-storage of unfertilized mouse eggs. Fertil Steril 10:384–396

Trounson A (1984) In vitro fertilization and embryo preservation. In: Trounson A, Wood C (eds) In vitro fertilization and embryo transfer. Churchill Livingstone, Edinburgh, pp 111–130

Van Uem JFHM, Siebzehnrubl ER, Schuh B, Koch R, Trotnow S, Lang N (1987) Birth after cryopreservation of unfertilized oocytes. Lancet I:752–753

Whittingham DG (1977) Fertilization in vitro and development to term of unfertilized mouse oocytes previously stored at −196 °C. J Reprod Fertil 49:89–94

10 Embryo Cryopreservation

A. Trounson

10.1 Introduction

Cryopreservation of mammalian embryos was initiated in 1972 by the independent experiments of Wilmut (1972) and Whittingham et al. (1972). These studies showed that the slow cooling of early cleavage stage mouse embryos to low sub-zero temperatures in the presence of dimethyl sulphoxide (DMSO) and slow warming during the thawing phase, resulted in the survival of embryos and their development to term. Embryos of many other species have been frozen using minor modifications of this technique. Human pre-implantation stage embryos were first successfully cryopreserved by Trounson and Mohr (1983) using a variation of this method and this has resulted in the introduction of embryo cryopreservation into clinical in vitro fertilization (IVF) (Mohr et al. 1985; Trounson 1986) as a way of dealing with the problem of excess embryos (Trounson et al. 1982). Cryopreservation also increases the chance of pregnancy for IVF patients (Fehilly et al. 1985; Trounson 1986) and is an option chosen most frequently by couples in the circumstances of having produced more oocytes or embryos than is required for replacement in the cycle of IVF treatment.

The method of slow cooling embryos is based on the need to avoid intracellular ice formation by progressive dehydration of cells during the ice-forming phase. The cryoprotective solutions used to freeze embryos are normally seeded around $-5\,°C$ to $-7\,°C$ by the introduction of ice crystals into the solution, or by touching the vial or straw containing the embryos with a metal instrument cooled in liquid nitrogen causing ice growth at the point of contact. Progressive slow cooling (less than 1 °C/minute) from the seeding temperature enables the growth of large rounded crystals of ice, drawing water out of the supercooling cells of the embryo as the salt concentration rises in the extracellular solution surrounding the embryos. Intracellular water diffusing out of the embryo is frozen and the extracellular salt concentrations continue to rise. The eutectic point for the major salt, sodium chloride, is $-21.5\,°C$ but it is possible that the high salt concentration in the extracellular solution surrounding the dehydrating embryos supercools to lower temperatures ($-30\,°C$ to $-40\,°C$) before crystallization occurs. Dehydration of the embryonic blastomeres reduces the chance of intracellular ice formation, considered lethal to the cell.

At temperatures around $-30\,°C$ to $-40\,°C$ embryos may be rapidly cooled to $-196\,°C$ by transfer to liquid nitrogen (Willadsen 1977; Whittingham et al. 1979), but they need to be thawed rapidly for cells to survive. It is presumed that rapid warming avoids growth of any small ice crystals formed because of incomplete dehydration during thawing. Embryos slow cooled to low sub-zero temperatures (below $-60\,°C$) need to be thawed slowly ($5-15\,°C/minute$) in order to prevent damaging osmotic effects on the dehydrated cell. Using these principles, embryos of many different species have been successfully cryopreserved.

It is essential to use a cryoprotectant for freezing to enable cells to survive. These chemicals have high hydrogen bonding capacity but their specific action in the cell during freezing and thawing is not well understood. The three main cryoprotectants used are DMSO, glycerol and 1,2-propanediol. Other chemicals such as methanol have cryoprotective properties but are not widely used. Protein is also usually added to the solution to enhance embryo survival (Harrison et al. 1987). The basic salt solution normally used is phosphate buffered saline (e.g. Dulbecco's phosphate buffered saline) or embryo culture media containing HEPES organic buffer (e.g. M2 medium – Quinn et al. 1982). Inadequately buffered culture media change pH quite dramatically during cooling, exposing embryos to excessively acid or alkaline conditions which may adversely affect their viability.

10.2   Requirements for Embryo Freezing

For conventional freezing techniques specific training and equipment is necessary (see Trounson and Freemann 1987). For slow cooling to sub-zero temperatures biological freezing machines are generally used. These instruments vary in cost depending on how much automation is desired, the accuracy of cooling required and the temperature to which controlled cooling is needed. In many cases they are excessively expensive and difficult to maintain. Many biological freezers require liquid nitrogen but if cooling to only $-30\,°C$ to $-40\,°C$ is needed electrical freezers may be used. In addition, liquid nitrogen storage facilities are required and these need to have automatic maintenance of liquid nitrogen levels or constant supervision in order to maintain the embryo bank.

The training of embryologists in freezing by conventional slow cooling techniques is critical. Poor results are frequently reported by untrained staff, and even in experienced IVF clinics difficulties have been encountered in successfully freezing human embryos. It is essential that repeatable success in freezing 2- to 8-cell mouse embryos be demonstrated by embryologists initiating human embryo freezing. The importance of this experience cannot be understated. Unfortunately biological freezers are subject to breakdown so that the embryologist needs to be in the near vicinity in order to rescue embryos and, importantly, to know what to do when this happens. For these reasons cryopreservation by slow cooling can be expensive in the equipment required and the embryologist's time. These costs are usually transferred to the patients, making it essential that success rates be maintained.

The embryos are normally thawed during the patient's spontaneous ovulatory cycle and it is therefore a requirement that the day of the luteinizing hormone (LH) surge, or day of ovulation, be accurately determined (see Trounson et al. 1983). The patient is normally monitored for endocrine changes indicative of ovulation (oestrogen and LH levels) or for follicular growth and ovulation by ultrasound. It is important to establish progesterone secretion from the corpus luteum before thawing and transfer of embryos (see Freemann et al. 1986). Coordination of the patient and of embryo thawing for replacement is usually done by the clinical and nursing staff of the IVF programme.

10.3   Development of Slow Cooling Methods for Cryopreserving Human Embryos

The initial studies on human embryo freezing (Trounson and Mohr 1983) utilized the slow cooling methods developed for successfully freezing cattle embryos (Trounson et al. 1978). We studied the cryoprotectants DMSO and glycerol, passing embryos stepwise through increasing concentrations of the cryoprotectants in Dulbecco's phosphate buffered saline containing 10% fetal calf serum or human serum. The embryos were sealed in glass ampoules, cooled to −7 °C at 2 °C/minute, seeded at −7 °C and slow cooled (0.1–0.3 °C/minute) to either −40 °C or −80 °C, then transferred to storage in liquid nitrogen. The embryos were thawed either rapidly in a warm water bath or slowly (8 °C/minute) depending on the final temperature reached during slow cooling. Embryo survival was highest when embryos were slow cooled in 1.5 M DMSO to low sub-zero temperatures (−80 °C or lower) and pregnancies were obtained using this method (Trounson and Mohr 1983). We observed that the permeability of glycerol into early cleavage stage human embryos was very slow and this cryoprotectant also induced cell fusion of adjacent blastomeres. The initial pregnancies obtained with human embryo cryopreservation by slow cooling in DMSO were restricted to early cleavage stage (4- to 16-cell) embryos (Trounson and Mohr 1983; Zeilmaker et al. 1984; Mohr et al. 1985; Freemann et al. 1986).

In the commercial cattle embryo transfer industry, cryopreservation has been concentrated on the blastocyst stage of development because this is the stage at which recovery is by non-surgical embryo flushing of the uterus. The freezing method used most frequently has been slow cooling in the cryoprotectant glycerol to relatively high sub-zero temperatures of −30 °C to −40 °C before storage in liquid nitrogen. Embryos are thawed rapidly in warm water-baths. The glycerol was usually added and removed stepwise through graded solutions. This technique was introduced into human IVF by R. F. Simons for freezing human blastocysts when he moved from the cattle industry to Bourn Hall and obtained pregnancies when thawed blastocysts were later replaced in utero (Cohen et al. 1985, 1986). This technique requires that human embryos be cultured to the blastocyst stage in vitro and has been reported to be highly successful (Fehilly et al. 1985). However, the method has not been widely adopted by other IVF clinics probably because of the extended time required to culture embryos to the blastocyst stage of development and the difficulty encountered in growing a high proportion of embryos to blastocysts.

The use of 1,2-propanediol as the cryoprotectant for early cleavage stage embryos was introduced by French scientists (Lasalle et al. 1985). This method also involves slow cooling of embryos to low sub-zero temperatures and uses sucrose in addition to the cryoprotective solution. Good results have been obtained using this cryoprotectant for freezing fertilized 1-cell pronuclear oocytes to 4-cell embryos (Testart et al. 1986) and is widely used in IVF for cryopreservation of human embryos.

At the present time, embryo cryopreservation using DMSO, 1,2-propanediol or occasionally glycerol is used in many IVF programmes in order to preserve excess embryos for the patients. While there is no general agreement about which slow cooling method is the best, it is probable that success rates of cryopreservation may depend more on the quality and viability of embryos produced in the individual IVF programme than on the method used for freezing. The close association of pregnancy in the cycle of IVF treatment and pregnancy after thawing the same batch of embryos (Freemann et al. 1986; Trounson 1986) supports this conclusion. Cryopreservation is a valuable addition to a highly successful IVF programme but is probably of little assistance for IVF programmes with low success rates.

10.4 Methods of Cryopreservation by Slow Cooling

10.4.1 Slow Cooling in DMSO

The solutions for slow cooling in DMSO cryoprotectant are usually prepared in Dulbecco's phosphate buffered saline (PBI) or M2 medium (Table 10.1). These solutions contain protein in the form of bovine or human serum albumin (BSA or HSA, Fraction V) but may also be supplemented with 10%–20% serum (fetal calf serum or human serum). These solutions are normally prepared in our own laboratory but Dulbecco's phosphate buffered saline may be purchased from commercial sources without protein and antibiotics. These need to be added before use in freezing. DMSO is added to PB1 or M2 and we normally prepare a 3 M DMSO solution (2.2 ml of DMSO in 7.8 ml of PB1 or M2) and store this solution at 4 °C before use. Graded solutions of 0, 0.25, 0.5, 1.0 and 1.5 M DMSO are prepared from the 3 M DMSO solution by mixing with PB1 or M2 in the appropriate proportions. The embryos are passed through these solutions by pipetting, at 5–10 minute intervals. The embryos are placed in tissue culture washed glass vials or ampoules, insemination straws or plastic freezing tubes. The embryos are then cooled to −7 °C (2 °C/minute), and ice formation initiated (seeding) at −7 °C by touching the vial, straw or tube with an instrument precooled in liquid nitrogen. Some biological freezers have automatic seeding devices and some straws are made with a chemical which induces ice formation at around −5 °C to −10 °C. The presence of ice at −7 °C needs to be checked after seeding before cooling is continued to lower temperatures. The exposure of

Table 10.1. Composition of ionic media used to prepare cryoprotective solutions

Phosphate buffered saline		Medium M2	
Chemical	Concentration (g/l)[a]	Chemical	Concentration (g/l)[a]
NaCl	8.00	NaCl	5.533
KCl	0.20	KCl	0.356
Na$_2$HPO$_4$	1.15	KH$_2$PO$_4$	0.162
KH$_2$PO$_4$	0.20	MgSO$_4$.7H$_2$O	0.293
MgCl$_2$.6H$_2$O	0.10	NaHCO$_3$	0.349
Glucose	1.00	HEPES	4.969
Kanamycin sulphate	0.025	Na lactate	2.610
		Na pyruvate	0.036
Phenol red	0.0025	Glucose	1.000
Bovine serum		Penicillin G	0.060
Albumin (fraction V)	4.00	Streptamycin sulphate	0.050
CaCl$_2$.2H$_2$O	0.1324[b]	Phenol red	0.010
		Bovine serum	
		Albumin (fraction V)	4.000
		CaCl$_2$.2H$_2$O	0.252[b]

[a] Pure water.
[b] Dissolved separately.

embryos to intense cold during seeding should be avoided and ice nucleation should be induced some distance from the embryos.

Slow cooling (0.3 °C/minute) in a biological freezer should be accurately controlled from −7 °C to −30 °C but is normally continued to −40 °C, then the embryos are plunged into liquid nitrogen (Zeilmaker et al. 1984) or cooled slowly to −80 °C and then more quickly (10 °C/minute) to −110 °C before storage in liquid nitrogen (Trounson and Mohr 1983; Trounson 1986). Our own studies have been more successful with slow cooling to −80 °C.

Once the embryos are in liquid nitrogen storage they should remain submerged under the liquid surface to avoid accidental warming. Under liquid nitrogen, embryos could probably be preserved indefinitely without risk of damage. However, local regulation or legislation may limit the time of storage for human embryos. In our own laboratory embryos have been stored for up to 6 years and they appear to be preserved as well as those kept for shorter periods, which is similar to observations of mouse embryos in long-term cryostorage (Glenister and Lyon 1986).

If slow cooling is terminated at −30 °C to −40 °C, embryos should be thawed rapidly (Willadsen 1977) by transferring the straw or ampoule from liquid nitrogen to a warm water bath (30 °C to 37 °C). If slow cooling is terminated at lower temperatures, embryos should be thawed slowly (8–10 °C/minute) from −80 °C to around 0 °C. During melting of ice it is important to mix the cryoprotective solution in order to prevent exposure of embryos to very high concentrations of DMSO which may layer out in the ampoule or straw during this phase of thawing.

Embryos are expelled into 1.5 M DMSO in PB1 with 10%–20% serum and then transferred through 1.25 M, 1.0, 0.75, 0.5, 0.25 and PB1 with serum at 6–10 minute intervals. The survival of embryos can be assessed during removal of DMSO and embryos are placed in culture at 37 °C until ready for replacement in utero. In our laboratory we normally only replace embryos with more than 50%

of their original cell numbers intact after thawing. We also limit the number of embryos replaced to a maximum of three.

10.4.2 Slow Cooling in 1,2-Propanediol

The cryoprotectant 1,2-propanediol is made up in phosphate buffered saline containing 20% human serum. Embryos are placed in phosphate buffered saline with serum and then transferred to 1.5 M 1,2-propanediol for 15 minutes. The embryos are then transferred to another 1.5 M 1,2-propanediol solution containing 0.1 M sucrose, drawn into an insemination straw, the straw sealed and then cooled to −7 °C at 2 °C/minute. The straws are seeded at −7 °C, slow cooled to −30 °C at 0.3 °C/minute and then cooled rapidly (50 °C/minute) to −190 °C before transfer into liquid nitrogen. Embryos are thawed rapidly (300 °C/minute) by transferring the insemination straw from liquid nitrogen to a water-bath at 20 °C for 40 seconds. The straws are then placed in a 30 °C water-bath and the embryos expelled into phosphate buffered saline containing 20% human serum, 1.0 M 1,2-propanediol and 0.2 M sucrose for 5 minutes. The 1,2-propanediol is removed in 0.5 M steps (two solutions) of 5 minutes and the sucrose removed finally in one step. Embryos with more than half of their original cells are replaced in utero, without prolonged culture in vitro, 0–3 hours after thawing (Testart et al. 1986). Embryo replacement is timed for the stage of development by identifying the day of the LH surge from daily blood samples, calculating the day of ovulation and adding the appropriate time for embryo development.

10.4.3 Slow Cooling in Glycerol

Glycerol may be made up in phosphate buffered saline or HEPES buffered culture medium containing 10%–20% human serum. No details of the basic freezing solution are given by Cohen et al. (1985) except that they state embryos were frozen in culture medium, presumably 5% CO_2 equilibrated Earle's medium with human serum. Five solutions of 1%, 2%, 4%, 6% and 8% (v/v) glycerol in culture medium are prepared and embryos are passed through these solutions at 10 minute intervals at ambient temperature. The embryos are transferred to glass ampoules containing 8% glycerol in culture medium and cooled to −7 °C at 1 °C/minute, the solution seeded and then cooled in a biological freezer to −36 °C at 0.3 °C/minute. The embryos are then transferred to liquid nitrogen for storage. Thawing is done by transferring the glass ampoule from nitrogen to a water-bath at 30 °C, stirring the ampoule to increase the warming rate. Glycerol is removed stepwise by pipetting the embryos through solutions of 8% glycerol for 10 minutes, 6% for 12 minutes, 5% for 14 minutes, 4% for 16 minutes, 3% for 18 minutes, 2% for 20 minutes and 1% for 20 minutes. The embryos are then washed twice in culture medium and warmed slowly to 37 °C and kept in culture until the blastocysts re-expand (2–20 hours in vitro). It is apparently important to thaw and replace frozen blastocysts on day 4 following ovulation because Cohen et al. (1986) report that blastocysts thawed and transferred on days 3 and 5 do not result in pregnancy.

On the menstrual cycle of embryo replacement, patients may be clomiphene-treated or untreated (Cohen et al. 1986) and the time of ovulation determined by the detection of the onset of the LH surge or by the administration of human chorionic gonadotrophin. While it is not clear what is meant by day 4 after ovulation, it would be presumed that the day of ovulation is day 0.

10.5   Success of Cryopreservation by Slow Cooling

It is difficult to determine the success rate of cryopreservation accurately from articles published to date because much of the data are selected for presentation of experimental results. The results in our own IVF programme involving the slow cooling of 2- to 8-cell embryos in DMSO is shown in Table 10.2. From this unselected data nine births or ongoing pregnancies (more than 16 weeks) were obtained in the year. This represents 7% of patients with frozen embryos or 11% of those transferred frozen embryos. This is proportionally a very small addition to the overall success rate of IVF (Table 10.3). Using a similar procedure with DMSO, Van Steirtegham et al. (1987) reported a pregnancy rate per transfer of 15% (9/62 patients) from frozen–thawed 2- to 8-cell embryos. They obtained a higher pregnancy rate per transfer of 23% (11/48 patients) when freezing mostly 1-cell pronucleate oocytes in 1,2-propanediol. These are good results for success rate per transfer on the survival rates of frozen embryos were 51% in both DMSO and 1,2-propanediol. There was no data given on the number of patients who had embryos thawed in this study. However, there appears to be some advantage in success rate of freezing pronuclear oocytes in 1,2-propanediol. It is possible that

Table 10.2. Summary of cryopreservation results at Monash IVF programme in 1987 using slow cooling in DMSO

	Number	Percentage
Patients who had embryos thawed	136	—
Embryos thawed	272	—
Embryos surviving[a]	115	42
Patients transferred embryos	81	60
Patients pregnant	11	14
Ongoing or delivered pregnancies	9	11

[a] With more than 50% of original cells intact.

Table 10.3. IVF results in Monash IVF programme in 1987 with fresh and frozen embryos

	Number	Percentage
Patients admitted for IVF treatment	1111	
Patients undergoing oocyte recovery	942	85
Patients transferred embryos	788	84
Pregnancies from fresh embryo transfers	123	16
Pregnancies from frozen embryo transfer	11	1
Total number of pregnancies	134	17

pronuclear-stage oocytes have a higher survival rate after freezing than cleavage stage embryos, irrespective of the freezing method used. In the data reported by Testart et al. (1986), the highest survival rate was observed with pronuclear oocytes (88%) and survival rate progressively declined with increasing cleavage divisions to the point of no survival at the 8- to 16-cell stage. In their study, 32 patients were transferred frozen–thawed embryos of less than 8-cells resulting in 10 pregnancies, 7 of which could be attributed with certainty to frozen–thawed embryos. The pregnancy rate of 22%–31% per transfer is excellent but no information was available on birth rates or the original number of patients who had embryos frozen. The information from these studies indicates that the freezing of pronuclear oocytes in 1,2-propanediol may produce better results than the freezing of cleavage-stage embryos in either 1,2 propanediol or DMSO. The slight bias in favour of pronuclear oocytes may occur when the better quality cleavage-stage embryos are chosen for transfer in the cycle of IVF, leaving poorer quality embryos for cryopreservation.

Mandelbaum et al. (1987) used 1.5 M propanediol to freeze 480 2- to 10-cell embryos and found that 0.1 M sucrose in the freezing medium (Lassalle et al. 1985) significantly increased survival of embryos after thawing to 61% compared with 46% without sucrose. They reported 33 pregnancies from 165 embryo replacement cycles (20%) when freezing in 1,2-propanediol and sucrose compared with 2 pregnancies from 20 replacement cycles (10%) when freezing in 1,2-propanediol alone. The cryoprotective solutions were made up in B2 culture medium (Api-System, Montalieu-Vercieu, France). They also found no difference in pregnancy rate when frozen–thawed embryos were transferred to spontaneous ovulatory cycles, those stimulated with fertility drugs and those in which patients were given steroid replacement therapy to stimulate an artificial menstrual cycle for egg donation. The cleavage stage of the embryos had no effect on embryo survival or viability. These results indicate that freezing of early cleavage stage embryos in 1,2-propanediol and sucrose is a good method for cryopreservation.

In a comparative study of the success rate of the cryopreservation of cleaving embryos (5- to 10-cell) and blastocysts reported by Fehilly et al. (1985), three ongoing pregnancies were obtained when cleaving embryos of 26 patients were thawed (12%), compared with seven pregnancies from cryopreserved blastocysts of 23 patients (30%). The cleaving embryos were slow cooled in DMSO and the blastocysts slow cooled in glycerol. The results of freezing blastocysts in glycerol are very good. However, updated results from the same clinic reported by Ashwood-Smith (1986) show that 18 pregnancies have been obtained from 108 patients transferred embryos (17%), which indicates there has been a substantial decrease in the initial success rate reported. Considering the attrition rate of embryos developing to the blastocyst stage in vitro, it appears there may be little advantage in freezing blastocysts, except that cryopreservation would be needed less frequently than for pronuclear oocytes or early cleavage stage embryos.

Other reports contain too few patients to properly assess success rates of cryopreservation. For example, Zeilmaker et al. (1984) and Lucena et al. (1986) reported two births and one ongoing pregnancy, respectively, using slow cooling to $-39\,°C$ to $-40\,°C$ in 1.5 M DMSO. These pregnancies were obtained with small numbers of patients. Quinn and Kerin (1986) reported two ongoing pregnancies from 29 patients in which embryos were thawed and seven patients transferred embryos. Four of the patients had their embryos vitrified and one patient was transferred embryos surviving vitrification. Embryos from the other patients were slow cooled to $-80\,^\circ$C in 1.5 M DMSO.

10.6   The Development of Rapid Cooling Methods for Cryopreservation

10.6.1   Vitrification

Interest has developed in rapid freezing techniques for pre-implantation embryos. One approach which has received a lot of attention is vitrification, where concentrated solutions of cryoprotectants solidify or form glass instead of crystals. This glass is more like a very viscous, supercooled liquid than the crystalline form of frozen solutions. Vitrification has certain advantages over freezing because it may avoid the damage caused by intracellular ice formation and the osmotic effects caused by extracellular ice formation (Rall 1987).

Vitrification of cleavage stage mouse embryos was first reported by Rall and Fahy (1985) using high concentrations of DMSO, acetamide, 1,2-propanediol and polyethylene glycol. The total content of these solutes needs to be in excess of 40% (v/v) in order to enable the cryoprotective solution to vitrify during rapid cooling. These solutions are toxic to cells at ambient temperature, so embryos are placed in the final vitrification solutions at low temperatures (0 $^\circ$C to 4 $^\circ$C). Even though survival of embryos after vitrification was high, viability of embryos in vivo was not as good as that obtained by slow cooling methods (Rall et al. 1985, 1987). Changes to solute composition of the vitrification solution have reduced the toxicity to mouse embryos at 4 $^\circ$C, particularly a solution composed of 6.5 M glycerol and 6% polyethylene glycol (Rall 1987).

Embryos need to be partially dehydrated for vitrification and they are normally equilibrated in a stepwise procedure by exposure to 25% strength of the final vitrification solution at room temperature until the cryoprotectants have fully permeated the cells (20–30 minutes). Embryos are then placed in 50% strength of the vitrification medium for 10 minutes at 4 $^\circ$C and finally into the full strength vitrification solution for 10 minutes at 4 $^\circ$C before drawing them into insemination straws, sealing the straws and plunging them into liquid nitrogen. Embryos are thawed by transferring straws from liquid nitrogen to a cold bath (0 $^\circ$C to 4 $^\circ$C) and the cryoprotective solutes removed stepwise in 10 minute steps in 50% and 25% strength vitrification solution at 4 $^\circ$C, and 10 minute steps in 25%, 12.5% and 0% (isotonic saline) at room temperature (22 $^\circ$C). An alternative to this lengthy stepwise procedure is to transfer embryos directly from full strength vitrification solution into saline containing 1.04 M sucrose at 4 $^\circ$C for 5 minutes, a further 5 minutes at room temperature, and then to isotonic saline for 10 minutes (Rall 1987). The permeating cryoprotective solutes are removed in the sucrose solution without causing excessive swelling of the cells. Water is replaced when the embryos are transferred from the sucrose solution into isotonic saline, thus returning the cells to its original volume.

One of the unusual components of the original vitrifying solutions was acetamide, which was introduced to reduce the chemical toxicity of DMSO.

However, acetamide is a weak carcinogen and we have observed (Kola et al. 1988) fetal malformations after exposing unfertilized mouse oocytes to vitrifying solutions. Removal of the high concentrations of acetamide from the vitrifying solutions would be advisable and new vitrifying solutions which do not contain acetamide or DMSO are now in use (Rall 1987).

Scheffen and colleagues (1988) have used a combination of 25% glycerol and 25% 1,2-propanediol (v/v) in phosphate buffered saline as the vitrification solution. Embryos are equilibrated in a solution containing 10% glycerol and 20% 1,2-propanediol at ambient temperature for 10 minutes and then loaded quickly in a drop (20 μg) of vitrification solution (25% glycerol and 25% 1,2-propanediol in phosphate buffered saline) in an insemination straw (0.25 ml). The vitrification solution is separated by two air bubbles from dilution solutions of 1 M sucrose in phosphate buffered saline which fills the remainder of the straw. The straw is then plunged progressively into liquid nitrogen within 30 seconds in order not to cause mixing of the sucrose dilution solution and the vitrification solution. Embryos are thawed by shaking in a warm water-bath (20 °C), mixing the sucrose and vitrification solutions. The mixed solution is left for 5 minutes at ambient temperature and then the embryos are washed three times in phosphate buffered saline before culture in vitro or transfer to recipients. This is a simpler method of vitrification and retains high viability of morulae and early blastocysts in vitro and in vivo. The results for vitrification of expanding blastocysts were poor.

10.6.2 Vapour Freezing

A number of researchers have examined rapid freezing methods using high concentrations of glycerol. Miyamoto and Ishibashi (1986) added glycerol in two increments at 10 minute intervals to mouse embryos in phosphate buffered saline at 0 °C to a final concentration of 2 M. Embryos were held in 2 M glycerol for 10 minutes then placed in liquid nitrogen vapour for 10–15 minutes before being immersed in liquid nitrogen. Embryos were rapidly thawed in a 40 °C water-bath and transferred to phosphate buffered saline containing 2 M glycerol and 0.5 M sucrose for 3 minutes, then phosphate buffered saline containing 0.5 M sucrose for 3 minutes at room temperature before washing twice in phosphate buffered saline and being placed in culture. In their studies, survival rate of embryos was higher in 2 M glycerol than in 2 M 1,2-propanediol or 2 M ethylene glycol and was substantially higher than in 2 M DMSO. No difference was observed between embryos pretreated or not with 0.5 M sucrose. On the other hand, Szell and Shelton (1986) found that a freezing solution of 3 M glycerol and 0.25 M sucrose prepared in phosphate buffered saline with 5% fetal calf serum gave optimum results. Embryos were equilibrated in 40 μl 3 M glycerol and 0.25 M sucrose for 10 minutes at room temperature in insemination straws. The remainder of the straw was filled with a sucrose diluent (0.5–1.0 M sucrose in phosphate buffered saline) and separated from the freezing solution containing the embryos by a small air bubble. Straws were sealed and placed horizontally in liquid nitrogen vapour for 7–10 minutes before submerging them in liquid nitrogen. Embryos were thawed in a 35 °C water-bath, mixing the embryos in the freezing medium with sucrose diluent and allowing them to equilibrate to 10 minutes at 20 °C before pipetting into phosphate buffered saline for a further 10–20 minutes and culture in vitro.

These researchers reported later (Szell and Shelton 1987) that addition of glycerol and sucrose in two steps (3–4 M glyceerol for 5 minutes then glycerol and 0.5 M sucrose for 5 minutes) was better than one step. High rates of development of frozen–thawed 8- to 16-cell embryos to blastocysts was obtained and in a small study development in vivo was close to that of non-frozen embryos if cultured for 24 hours in vitro before transferring to foster mothers. Bovine embryos have also been successfully frozen using a similar method in 2.1 M glycerol and 0.25 M sucrose (Chupin 1987).

10.6.3   Ultrarapid Freezing

A very simple snap freezing method has been developed by Trounson et al. (1987) which uses 3–4 M DMSO and 0.25 M sucrose in phosphate buffered saline or HEPES buffered M2 medium containing bovine serum albumin (BSA) as the freezing solution. Embryos are pipetted directly into about 40 μl of this solution in an insemination straw for 2.5–3.0 minutes, the straw sealed and then plunged directly into liquid nitrogen. Embryos are thawed in a 37 °C water-bath and expelled into 0.125–0.25 M sucrose in phosphate buffered saline or M2 for 5–10 minutes to remove the DMSO and then cultured in vitro or transferred to recipients. In the original study (Trounson et al. 1987) the viability of frozen–thawed 2-cell mouse embryos in vitro and in vivo was equal to that obtained by slow cooling to low sub-zero temperatures (-80 °C) in 1.5 M DMSO. Exposure of embryos to the freezing solutions had no effect on the viability of embryos. The success of the method was confirmed with 8-cell mouse embryos (Trounson et al. 1988) and it was shown that despite similar rates of development to blastocysts in vitro, freezing in 3.5 M DMSO was significantly better for viability in vivo than freezing in 2.0 M DMSO. Fetal development of 8-cell embryos frozen in 3.5 M DMSO was not significantly different to that of non-frozen controls. The reduced viability of embryos frozen in 2.0 M DMSO could be explained by a significant reduction of cell numbers in blastocysts due to either undetected damage of some blastomeres during freezing or a reduction in cell cleavage rate. This reduction in cell numbers at the blastocyst stage probably accounts for the increased proportion of implanting blastocysts which do not continue normal development to fetuses when embryos are frozen in 2 M DMSO (Trounson et al. 1988). Further studies (J. M. Shaw and A. Trounson, unpublished) have shown that highly repeatable success rates can be achieved with ultrarapid freezing in 3 M DMSO with 0.25 M sucrose of protein concentrations are maintained (4–32 mg/ml BSA). Harrison et al. (1987) observed maximum viability in vitro was obtained when freezing solutions contained 4 mg/ml BSA when embryos were slow cooled in 1.5 M DMSO. We have also noted that during the 3 minute equilibration in DMSO and sucrose the straw should be kept still on the bench rather than agitated. This keeps the embryos on the inside surface of the straw rather than in the centre of the solution and this makes a substantial difference to embryo viability for some reason. In another study (Shaw et al. 1988) we found that irradiation of insemination straws for sterilization changes the surface properties of the plastic straws, increasing gas bubble formation and reducing embryo survival and development. Taking these precautions, survival rates of embryos after freezing and thawing exceed 90% and viability in vitro and in vivo is equivalent to that of non-frozen embryos.

The freezing method is so simple and quick, involves no expensive freezing machines and produces such good results with cleavage-stage mouse embryos, that it is likely to replace other methods of cryopreservation. It should be noted that this method is not suitable for freezing blastocyst-stage embryos and that some major modifications are necessary to enable high survival rates of these later stages of pre-implantation embryonic development.

10.7   Use of Rapid Freezing Methods for Cryopreservation of Human Embryos

The only report of vitrification of human embryos has been by Quinn and Kerin (1986). They vitrified 22 embryos and of 11 embryos warmed only one survived (9%). Vapour freezing of human embryos has not been reported to date.

Trounson et al. (1988) ultrarapidly froze 11 cleavage stage embryos from six patients in 2 M DMSO and 0.25–0.5 M sucrose. Nine of these embryos survived with more than 50% of their original cells intact (seven embryos were completely intact) but no pregnancies were obtained when the thawed embryos were replaced in utero in the six patients. In order to examine the capacity of human embryos to continue development in vitro, Trounson and Sjöblom (1988) ultrarapidly froze all the excess embryos from the Gothenburg IVF programme and cultured them in vitro after thawing. The embryos were frozen in 3 M DMSO and 0.25 M sucrose in phosphate buffered saline with 4 mg/ml BSA. Of 20 embryos ranging from a pronuclear oocyte to 8- to 12-cell embryos 85% survived and 88% continued cleavage after thawing. Two of the 17 surviving embryos developed to blastocysts. We also noted that fewer embryos frozen in freshly prepared DMSO solutions (embryos frozen within 1 hour of preparing the solution) survived freezing (50%) when compared with embryos frozen in solutions prepared 24–72 hours before freezing (94%). On the basis of these results we have begun clinical trials using the ultrarapid freezing technique.

10.8   Cryopreservation of Embryos and Unfertilized Oocytes

There is a desire to develop cryopreservation techniques for unfertilized oocytes as an alternative to fertilized oocytes and early cleavage stage embryos. The perceived ethical advantages of freezing unfertilized oocytes must be considered along with the disadvantages to the patients and the possible increased risks of oocyte freezing compared with that of embryos.

Fertilization rates in human IVF average around 70% of oocytes inseminated. However, the range for patients is 0–100%. When freezing oocytes a decision has to be made about the number inseminated and the number frozen before the actual number of oocytes fertilized is known. It is strongly recommended that only three or four embryos be transferred at any one time, so if a clinic freezes only unfertilized oocytes a maximum of three to four oocytes will be inseminated and the remainder frozen. Since it is not possible to predict fertilization rate for any individual patient, the number of embryos replaced in the cycle of IVF treatment will be reduced by about 30% below that of IVF programmes that do not freeze oocytes or freeze embryos. The number of embryos transferred is the major factor controlling pregnancy rate (Wood et al. 1985), hence oocyte freezing reduces pregnancy rate for patients in their cycle of IVF treatment (Table 10.4). This reduction of IVF success rate needs to be recovered by increased pregnancies from frozen–thawed oocytes.

Table 10.4. Reduction in the number of pregnancies expected when freezing unfertilized oocytes if the number of oocytes inseminated is restricted to four[a]

No. of embryos transferred	Actual IVF data in 1985		Expected results if only 4 oocytes inseminated	
	No. of patients transferred embryos	No. of pregnancies	No. of patients transferred embryos	Expected no. of pregnancies
0	94	0	109	0
1	120	5	146	6
2	125	23	205	38
3	358	75	237	50
Total	697	103	697	93

[a] Assuming the same frequency of fertilization rate and pregnancy rate observed in the Monash IVF programme in 1985 (J. M. Shaw and A. Trounson, unpublished).

It would seem improbable that freezing unfertilized oocytes could be more successful than freezing fertilized oocytes or embryos. The reasons for this are firstly that any damage to the zona pellucida, even minute cracks not easily seen under the microscope, will radically increase polyspermy in the human. The same problem is not so obvious in mouse oocytes because in this species there is a substantial block to polyspermy at the vitelline membrane. There is no vitelline block to polyspermy in the human. A dramatic increase in polyploidy in frozen–thawed human oocytes was reported by Al-Hasani et al. (1987). When frozen by slow cooling in 1,2-propanediol and sucrose 40% of fertilized eggs were polyploid and in DMSO 20% of fertilized eggs were polyploid. Minor cracks to the zona in pronuclear oocytes or embryos has no effect on their viability. Secondly, any damage to the vitelline membrane of oocytes will destroy the oocyte completely, but even when some cells of a cleaved embryo are damaged, the embryo can continue normal development to term (Trounson and Mohr 1983; Freemann et al. 1986). Our own experiments of freezing unfertilized oocytes show that survival after thawing, fertilization and development is always much lower (Table 10.5) than survival and development of cleavage-stage embryos after freezing and thawing. Similar low success rates were reported for survival and fertilization of unfertilized human oocytes (Al-Hasani et al. 1987). Given these results it is difficult to imagine that viability of unfertilized oocytes could approach that of pronuclear oocytes or embryos after cryopreservation.

Concerns still exist about the safety of freezing the unfertilized oocyte which has chromosomes in a condensed state on the spindle of the second meiotic

Table 10.5. Survival and fertilization of unfertilized mouse oocytes frozen by slow cooling techniques[a]

Freezing method	Number of oocytes frozen	Percentage survived, fertilized and developed to 2-cells
Slow cooling to −36 °C		
DMSO added 22 °C	782	4%
DMSO added 0 °C[b]	621	3%
Slow cooling to −80 °C		
DMSO added 22 °C	416	16%
DMSO added 0 °C[c]	613	42%
Control (not frozen)	516	91%

[a] Data from C. Kirby and A. Trounson (unpublished data).
[b] Method used by Chen (1986) for freezing human oocytes.
[c] Method used by Glenister et al. (1987).

division. The spindle microtubules depolymerize during cooling (Pickering and Johnson 1987; Sathananthan et al. 1988) and may not repolymerize properly during warming, giving rise to chromosome scattering and micronuclei (Sathananthan et al. 1987). This may increase the chance of aneuploidy following fertilization. Glenister et al. (1987) found no increase in aneuploidy of frozen–thawed mouse oocytes but found an increase in polyspermy. However, Kola et al. (1988) found a three- to four-fold increase in aneuploidy after freezing by slow cooling in 1.5 M DMSO and after vitrification. We also observed fetal malformations after vitrifying mouse oocytes. An increase in aneuploidy would increase miscarriage and may increase birth defects. Given the present information we would recommend that freezing of unfertilized oocytes should be very carefully considered before being introduced into clinical IVF. Most IVF groups that were freezing unfertilized oocytes have now changed to freezing fertilized pronuclear oocytes.

Freezing cleavage-stage embryos during metaphase of the cell cycle may also result in chromosomal damage or loss but this is a very short phase of the normal cell cycle of embryonic cleavage stages. We would also advise embryologists in IVF not to freeze embryos around the time of cleavage, to avoid this potential hazard.

10.9   Conclusion

Cryopreservation has been widely incorporated into clinical IVF and is presently based on slow cooling methods using the cryoprotectants DMSO and 1,2-propanediol. There appears to be some advantage in success rates if pronuclear oocytes are frozen in 1,2-propanediol, with pregnancy rates of around 20%–25% of patients transferred embryos. Slow cooling of early cleavage stage embryos in DMSO results in pregnancy rates of 10%–15% of patients transferred embryos. Some IVF clinics may still freeze blastocysts in glycerol but it is difficult to determine success rates for this procedure.

New methods of rapid freezing have been developed using mouse embryos. These methods include vitrification, vapour freezing and ultrarapid freezing. It is too early to assess their value in human IVF but they are replacing slow cooling methods for cryopreserving animal embryos. These methods are quick and inexpensive and are potentially more successful than slow cooling methods.

The freezing of unfertilized oocytes should be evaluated carefully because of the likely reduced success rate, increased expense because it involves freezing more frequently, and the abnormalities observed in chromosomal number, polyspermy and, in the case of vitrification, fetal malformations. In view of these concerns it may be advisable to freeze pronuclear oocytes if ethical or legal restrictions are imposed on embryo freezing.

References

Al-Hasani S, Diedrich K, van der Ven H, Reinecke A, Hartje M, Krebs D (1987) Cryopreservation of human oocytes. Hum Reprod 2:695–700

Ashwood-Smith MJ (1986) The cryopreservation of human embryos. Hum Reprod 1:319–332

Chen C (1986) Pregnancy after human oocyte cryopreservation. Lancet I:884–886

Cohen J, Simons RF, Edwards RG, Fehilly CB, Fishel SB (1985) Pregnancies following the frozen storage of expanding human blastocysts. J In Vitro Fertil Embryo Transfer 2:59–64

Cohen J, Simons RF, Fehilly CB, Edward RG (1986) Factors affecting survival and implantation of cryopreserved human embryos. J In Vitro Fertil Embryo Transfer 3:46–52

Chupin D (1987) Quick freezing of day 7 bovine blastocysts: optimum parameters of dehydration step. Theriogenology 27:219

Fehilly CB, Cohen J, Simons RF, Fishel SB, Edwards RG (1985) Cryopreservation of cleaving embryos and expanded blastocysts in the human: a comparative study. Fertil Steril 44:638–644

Freemann L, Trounson A, Kirby C (1986) Cryopreservation of human embryos: progress on the clinical use of the technique in human in vitro fertilization. J In Vitro Fertil Embryo Transfer 3:53–61

Glenister PH, Lyon MF (1986) Long-term storage of eight-cell mouse embryos at −196°C. J In Vitro Fertil Embryo Transfer 3:20–27

Glenister PH, Wood MJ, Kirby C, Whittingham DG (1987) Incidence of chromosome anomalies in first-cleavage mouse embryos obtained from frozen–thawed oocytes fertilized in vitro. Gamete Res 16:205–216

Harrison KL, Pope AK, Wilson LM, Breen TM, Cummins JM (1987) The optimum concentration of albumin as an embryo cryoprotectant. J In Vitro Fertil Embryo Transfer 4:286–288

Kola I, Kirby C, Shaw J, Davey A, Trounson A (1988) Vitrification of mouse oocytes results in aneuploid zygotes and malformed fetuses. Teratology (in press)

Lassalle B, Testart J, Renard J-P (1985) Human embryo features that influence the success of cryopreservation with the use of 1,2-propanediol. Fertil Steril 44:645–651

Lucena E, Olivares R, Obando H et al. (1986) Pregnancies following transfer of human frozen–thawed embryos in Colombia, South America. Hum Reprod 1:383–385

Mandelbaum J, Junca AM, Plachot M et al. (1987) Human embryos cryopreservation, extrinsic and intrinsic parameters of success. Hum Reprod 2:709–715

Miyamoto H, Ishibashi T (1986) Liquid nitrogen vapour freezing of mouse embryos. J Reprod Fertil 78:471–478

Mohr LR, Trounson A, Freemann L (1985) Deep-freezing and transfer of human embryos. J In Vitro Fertil Embryo Transfer 2:1–10

Pickering SJ, Johnson MH (1987) The influence of coolu. ˜ on the organization of the meiotic spindle of the mouse oocyte. Hum Reprod 2:207–216

Quinn P, Kerin JFP (1986) Experience with the cryopreservation of human embryos using the mouse as a model to establish successful techniques. J in Vitro Fertil Embryo Transfer 3:40–45

Quinn P, Barros C, Whittingham DG (1982) Preservation of hamster oocytes to assay the fertilizing capacity of human spermatozoa. J Reprod Fertil 66:161–168

Rall WF (1987) Factors affecting the survival of mouse embryos cryopreserved by vitrification. Cryobiology 24:387–402

Rall WF, Fahy GM (1985) Ice-free cryopreservation of mouse embryos at −196 °C by vitrification. Nature 313:573–575

Rall WF, Wood MJ, Kirby C (1985) In vivo development of mouse embryos cryopreserved by vitrification. Cryobiology 22:603–604

Rall WF, Wood MJ, Kirby C, Whittingham DG (1987) Development of mouse embryos cryopreserved by vitrification. J Reprod Fertil 80:499–504

Sathananthan AH, Trounson A, Freemann L (1987) Morphology and fertilizability of frozen human oocytes. Gamete Res 16:343–354

Sathananthan AH, Trounson A, Freemann L, Brady T (1988) The effects of cooling human oocytes. Hum Reprod (in press)

Scheffen B, Van Der Zwalmen P, Massip A (1986) A simple and efficient procedure for preservation of mouse embryos by vitrification. Cryo-Letters 7:260–269

Shaw JM, Diotellevi L, Trounson A (1988) Ultrarapid embryo freezing: effect of dissolved gas and pH of the freezing solution and straw irradiation. Hum Reprod (in press)

Szell A, Shelton JN (1986) Sucrose dilution of glycerol from mouse embryos frozen rapidly in liquid nitrogen. J Reprod Fertil 76:401–408

Szell A, Shelton JN (1987) Osmotic and cryoprotective effects of glycerol–sucrose solutions on day-3 mouse embryos. J Reprod Fertil 80:309–316

Testart J, Lassalle B, Belaisch-Allart J et al. (1986) High pregnancy rate after early human embryo freezing. Fertil Steril 46:268–272

Trounson A (1986) Preservation of human eggs and embryos. Fertil Steril 46:1–12

Trounson A, Freemann L (1987) Role of cryopreservation of human oocytes and embryos in an IVF program. In: Behrman SJ, Kistner RW, Patton GW (eds) Progress in infertility. Little Brown, Boston, pp 621–629

Trounson A, Mohr L (1983) Human pregnancy following cryopreservation, thawing and transfer of an eight-cell embryo. Nature 305:707–709

Trounson A, Sjöblom P (1988) Cleavage and development of human embryos in vitro after ultrarapid freezing and thawing. Fertil Steril 50:373–376

Trounson AO, Shea BF, Ollis GW, Jacobson ME (1978) Frozen storage and transfer of bovine embryos. J Anim Sci 47:667–681

Trounson AO, Wood C, Leeton J (1982) Freezing of human embryos: an ethical obligation. Med J Aust 2:332–334

Trounson AO, Burger HG, Kovacs GT (1983) Prediction of ovulation for in vitro fertilization. In: Jeffcoate SL (ed) Ovulation: methods for its prediction and detection. John Wiley, Chichester, pp 83–102

Trounson A, Peura A, Kirby C (1987) Ultrarapid freezing: a new low-cost and effective method of embryo cryopreservation. Fertil Steril 48:843–850

Trounson A, Peura A, Freemann L, Kirby C (1988) Ultrarapid freezing of early cleavage stage human embryos and eight-cell mouse embryos. Fertil Steril 49:822–826

Van Steirteghem AC, Van de Abbeel E, Camus M et al. (1987) Cryopreservation of human embryos obtained after gamete intra-fallopian transfer and/or in vitro fertilization. Hum Reprod 2:593–598

Whittingham DG, Leibo SP, Mazur P (1972) Survival of mouse embryos frozen to −196 °C and −269 °C. Science 178:411–414

Whittingham DG, Wood MJ, Farrant J, Lee H, Halsey JA (1979) Survival of frozen mouse embryos after rapid thawing from −196 °C. J Reprod Fertil 56:11–21

Willadsen SM (1977) Factors affecting the survivial of sheep embryos during deep-freezing and thawing. In: Elliott K, Whelan J (eds) The freezing of mammalian embryos. Elsevier, Amsterdam, pp 175–189

Wilmut I (1972) The effect of cooling rate, warming rate of cryoprotective agent, and stage of development on survival of mouse embryos during freezing and thawing. Life Sci 11:1071–1079

Wood C, McMaster R, Rennie G, Trounson A, Leeton J (1985) Factors influencing pregnancy rates following in vitro fertilization and embryo transfer. Fertil Steril 43:245–250

Zeilmaker GH, Alberda AT, van Gent I, Rijkmans CMPM, Drogendijk AC (1984) Two pregnancies following transfer of intact frozen–thawed embryos. Fertil Steril 42:293–296

11   Oocyte Donation

P. A. W. Rogers, J. Leeton, I. T. Cameron, C. Murphy, D. L. Healy and P. Lutjen

11.1   Introduction

Oocyte donation, unlike its male counterpart of sperm donation which has been a routine clinical treatment for male infertility for many years, has only become feasible since the widespread introduction of in vitro fertilization (IVF). Prior to the advent of IVF there was neither a source of oocytes for donation nor the laboratory or clinical techniques available to ensure successful fertilization and transfer of the resulting embryo. There are now several reports in the literature of successful pregnancies following oocyte donation to patients either unwilling or unable to conceive from their own oocytes (Lutjen et al. 1984; Feichtinger and Kemeter 1985; Navot et al. 1986; Rosenwaks et al. 1986; Asch et al. 1987; Serhal and Craft 1987; Devroey et al. 1987). A number of variations in the clinical use of donated oocytes now exist. These include fertilization with husband or donor semen, transfer to recipients with or without endogenous ovarian function, and more recently, the use of gamete intra-fallopian transfer (GIFT) rather than IVF (Asch et al. 1987). In addition to providing an avenue for successful pregnancy in those patients with hypergonadotrophic hypogonadism or inheritable genetic disorders, oocyte donation also provides a unique opportunity for the study and understanding of the steroid replacement parameters necessary to induce uterine receptivity, the synchronization of embryo development with uterine receptivity prior to implantation, and the endocrinology of pregnancy in the absence of ovarian function.

11.2   Indications for Donor Oocytes

Women who require donor oocytes occur in two main groups:

1. Women with non-functioning ovaries:
   a) Premature menopause

  b) Ovarian agenesis
  c) Bilateral oophorectomy
2. Women with functioning ovaries:
  a) Risk of inheritable genetic disease in children
  b) Failed IVF due to oocyte abnormality

Prior to 1986 a third category of ovulatory women requiring oocyte donation comprised those patients whose ovaries were inaccessible to laparoscopic visualization and oocyte collection. The recent development of ultrasonic scanning of the ovaries, particularly by the vaginal approach, has made oocyte collection using ultrasound control possible for most cases with pelvic pathology (Lenz 1984; Lenz et al. 1987).

11.3 Clinical Management

11.3.1 Counselling

Counselling and assessment of each recipient couple participating in a donor oocyte programme is essential and should be undertaken by a trained social (or equivalent) worker who is independent of the medical management team. In cases where the donor is known to the recipient, it is important to counsel both the donor and recipient couples together as a foursome, and separately as a couple (Leeton and Harman 1987).

11.3.2 Synchronization

The synchronization of ovulation between oocyte donors and recipients is mandatory although the post-ovulatory "window" of cycle days in the recipient for achieving pregnancy has yet to be accurately defined (see Sect. 11.6). Synchronization of ovulation between oocyte donor and ovulating recipient was originally described by Trounson and colleagues (1983). Approximate synchronization of ovulation has also been achieved by extension of the donor's luteal phase (Templeton et al. 1984). Timing of ovulation in the recipient in our programme is made by 12-hourly tracking of plasma E_2 and luteinizing hormone (LH) to identify the onset of the LH surge (Trounson et al. 1983). The semen of the recipient's husband may be stored by deep-freezing so that it is available at short notice for IVF if an oocyte is collected (Mahadevan et al. 1983).

Synchronization of the oocyte donor's cycle and the non-ovulating recipient's steroid replacement has been aimed at transfer on approximately day 17 of the recipient's cycle, although a wider "window" between days 14 and 20 is now being studied. Synchronization of cycles between a known donor and non-ovulating recipient may be readily achieved by manipulating the recipient's dosage schedule in the month preceding the transfer cycle.

The storage of donor embryos by cryopreservation offers an easier method of synchronization between donor and recipient cycles than does manipulation of the patients' cycles for both ovulating and non-ovulating recipients. The effectiveness of frozen–thawed embryos in our hands, however, remains less than that of non-frozen embryos, and at present they are used only when synchronization proves impossible.

11.3.3 Embryo Transfer

The technique of embryo transfer has already been described (Leeton et al. 1982). No differences were noted in difficulty of transfer between the oocyte recipient group and routine patients on the IVF programme, despite the fact that non-ovulating recipients were all nulliparous and had smaller uteri.

11.4 Source of Donor Oocytes

11.4.1 IVF Patients

The primary source of donated oocytes has come from patients on the IVF programme who have "excess" oocytes collected. The policy of the Monash group has been to transfer a maximum of three embryos at any one procedure because of the significant risks associated with high multiple pregnancies. Oocytes in excess of three may be either fertilized in vitro with the husband's sperm and deep-frozen, donated to a matched recipient for IVF and embryo transfer, or donated for research purposes. The choice is made prior to treatment by the couple after several interviews over the long waiting period.

Surveys of the attitudes towards oocyte donation have shown that donation is made for unselfish reasons and payment is not expected; most donors had told others of their donation so that the keeping of records would appear essential for possible future identification (Leeton and Harman 1986). Anonymity is maintained between donor and recipient couples, although non-identifying information is available to both on request.

11.4.2 Known Donors

Because of the shortage of oocyte donors, some recipients seek their own donor who is either a close friend or relation. Additional counselling as a foursome is advisable because of the potential risk of the known donor identifying strongly with the resulting child, although initial surveys suggest that this is unlikely (Leeton and Harman 1987). The birth of a baby resulting from the donation of an oocyte by the sister of the recipient has been reported (Leeton et al. 1986a).

11.4.3 Volunteer Donors

Oocyte donors may be found who wish to provide anonymous infertile couples with their gametes for altruistic reasons, in the same way as sperm donation is made. The number we have encountered to date is small, because of the time needed for IVF stimulation and the relative invasiveness of the oocyte collection procedure.

11.4.4   Women Undergoing Sterilization

Oocyte donation may be made laparoscopically at the same time as sterilization. Our programme has found this group to be a disappointing source of donor oocytes (Leeton et al. 1986b).

11.4.5   Donation of Oocytes Fertilized In Vivo

This procedure, termed embryo flushing, is a well established technique in animal breeding. The first successful human pregnancy and delivery has been reported (Bustillo et al. 1984). An important ethical consideration is the risk of producing an unwanted pregnancy in the donor, either uterine or tubal, and for this reason the practice of this procedure in the human is unacceptable in Melbourne.

11.5   Steroid Replacement Therapy

Upon commencement of treatment at Monash, patients with hypergonadotrophic hypogonadism receive cyclic steroid replacement therapy (Lutjen et al. 1984, 1986). The replacement schedule consists of oestradiol valerate at 1 mg/day from days 1 to 5 and on days 27 and 28, 2 mg daily from days 6 to 9 and 14 to 26, and 6 mg daily from days 10 to 13. Progesterone is given as intravaginal suppositories commencing at 25 mg on the evening of day 15, 25 mg morning and evening on day 16, and 50 mg morning and evening from days 17 to 26. At the end of a 28-day cycle patients recommence at day 1.

The effectiveness of this steroid replacement therapy is assessed for all patients by measuring daily serum E_2 and P_4, and by taking a mid-secretory endometrial biopsy. Once appropriate serum E_2 and P_4 levels and endometrial histology have been established the patient is instructed to continue cyclical steroid replacement each month until an oocyte becomes available for donation. Following embryo transfer E_2 is maintained at 2 mg daily and progesterone at 50–100 mg daily for 12 days. If a serum beta-human chorionic gonadotrophin (β-hCG) is positive, steroid replacement is continued until after the luteo-placental shift. At this time the placental tissues become competent to maintain oestrogen and progesterone levels without the need for exogenous assistance (Csapo and Pulkkinen 1978).

Most other steroid replacement therapies for hypergonadotrophic hypogonadism follow the general format of that outlined above (e.g. Navot et al. 1986; Feichtinger and Kemeter 1985). In the latter case, replacement therapy was not cyclical, commencing only in the planned cycle of transfer. More recently two groups have demonstrated that it is possible to vary the length of the follicular phase and still obtain successful implantation and pregnancy (Serhal and Craft

1987; Asch et al. 1987). The first of these groups gave E_2 at 2 mg three or four times daily until it appeared that a donor oocyte would become available. The recipient then commenced P_4 at 100 mg daily the day prior to the donor oocytes being harvested. In the second case, Asch and co-workers gave E_2 at 6 mg daily from day 12 until donor oocytes became available. At this time the recipient received the donated oocytes and her husband's sperm by GIFT, and immediately commenced P_4 at 50 mg daily.

The apparent success of both these schedules demonstrates that the relative length of the oestrogen-dominated part of the follicular phase may not be overly important for the prospects of successful implantation. This matter is currently being further investigated. A second administrative advantage of this type of approach to replacement therapy is that recipients can be "held" for a number of days in the follicular phase while waiting for donor oocytes. This tactic greatly simplifies the problems of donor–recipient synchronization.

11.6   Uterine Receptivity for Implantation

Animal studies have demonstrated that the uterus is one of the few organs in the body capable of resisting invasion by the implanting embryo. Successful "implantation" in non-uterine tissues has been demonstrated on a number of occasions (Fawcett et al. 1947; Kirby 1963; Rogers et al. 1988), and can occur regardless of the sex or hormonal status of the recipient. The ability of the uterus to prevent implantation when asynchrony is deliberately engineered (Noyes and Dickman 1960) supports the notion that a uterine mechanism exists which is deleterious to embryonic survival, and that for successful implantation to occur this mechanism must be corrected. For commonly studied species such as laboratory rodents it has been hypothesized that three uterine states exist: an embryo hostile state, a neutral state and a receptive state (Psychoyos and Casimiri 1981). The neutral phase occurs during delayed implantation, and allows the blastocyst to reside in the uterine cavity in a dormant state for a variable length of time until maternal factors are suitable for implantation to proceed. At other times, similar blastocysts transferred to a hostile uterus will either degenerate or be expelled from the uterus within a few hours.

The mechanisms responsible for uterine hostility and receptivity are only poorly understood in well-researched species such as laboratory rodents, whilst almost nothing is known about them in the human. Although it has long been recognized that the human endometrium undergoes typical changes in structure as determined by light microscopic histology during the menstrual cycle (Noyes et al. 1950), it has not been possible to define any one appearance or group of characteristics that indicate receptivity for implantation. In fact, the only evidence that reduced uterine receptivity may play a role in preventing implantation in the human comes from statistical analysis of multiple pregnancy data generated by IVF programmes (Rogers et al. 1986; Walters et al. 1985). In these studies it has been estimated that reduced uterine receptivity following superovulation for IVF may be responsible for implantation failure in anything from 23% to 70% of cases. Despite the statistical nature of these estimates, and the wide

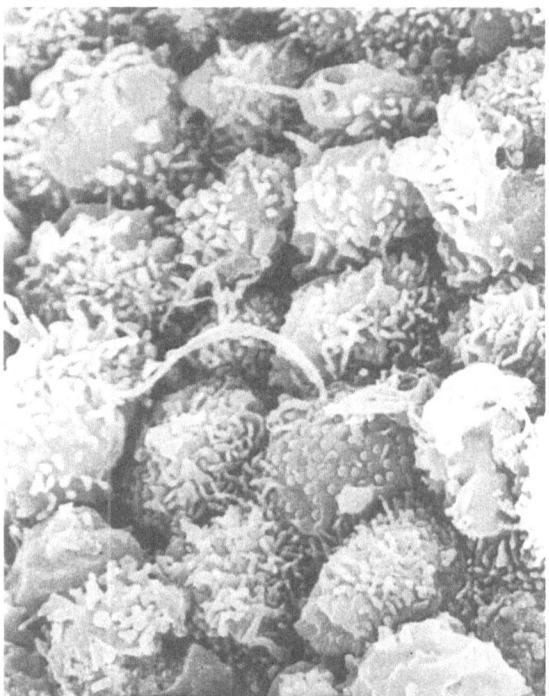

Fig. 11.1. Scanning electron micrograph (SEM) showing typical "receptive" epithelial cells from the uterus of a steroid replacement patient. In particular, note the short, irregular appearance of the microvilli, the bulging cell apices, and the appearance of other irregular protrusions. ($\times$ 5400)

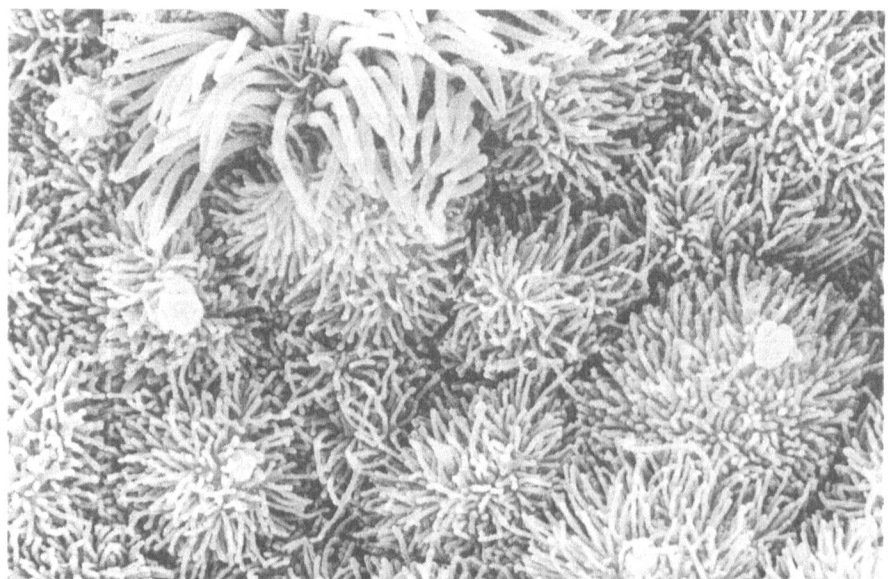

Fig. 11.2. SEM of "non-receptive" uterus showing long regular microvilli. (Ciliated cells are also present in this micrograph.) ($\times$ 5400)

variability in the results, the overall conclusion appears to be that in the human, as in most other mammals studied to date, the uterus is primarily responsible for controlling the success or failure of the implantation process, given a normal healthy embryo.

Notwithstanding the lack of information on uterine receptivity in the human, its clinical importance in contraceptive and infertility work, and the ethical and technical problems associated with research on human implantation, donor oocyte programmes for patients on steroid replacement therapy now represent an exciting new avenue for gaining further insights in this field. To date little serious advantage has been taken of this new opportunity for research, although this may be indicative of the general lack of basic knowledge from which to mount appropriate studies. In a recent ultrastructural study of endometrium taken from patients on steroid replacement therapy, the apical surface of uterine epithelial cells was described and a number of characteristics that may indicate receptivity were detailed (Murphy et al. 1987). Typical "receptive" and "non-receptive" appearances are shown in Figs. 11.1. and 11.2.

Studies currently in progress at Monash are aimed at describing further ultrastructural, histochemical, cell junction and membrane molecular biology changes, and correlating them to differing steroid replacement regimes. From these studies it will be possible to characterize the changing uterine parameters over the time when the uterus is believed to be receptive, and hopefully it will be possible to identify specific marker events that more closely define receptivity.

A review of the donor oocyte pregnancies achieved to date in women without ovarian function provides the first evidence of how wide the "window" of human uterine receptivity may be (Fig. 11.3). Not all authors quoted in Fig. 11.3 have published precise information as to the exact stage of embryonic development and the timing of transfer for each pregnancy. In such cases estimates have been deduced from the available data. The calculation of synchrony assumes that under natural conditions the uterus first "sees" significant progesterone 24 hours after the start of the LH surge, and that this is followed 12 hours later by ovulation, with fertilization commencing 6 hours after that. Thus the embryo becomes 2-cell 48 hours after the uterus first sees progesterone, 4-cell by 60 hours after progesterone, 8-cell by 72 hours and so on. The data in Fig. 11.3 are thus calculated as the difference in timing between the embryonic age at transfer and the elapsed time since the uterus first "saw" progesterone.

11.7   Endocrinology of Pregnancy

11.7.1   Luteo-placental Shift

The successful achievement of pregnancies resulting from the transfer of embryos derived from donated oocytes not only offers a realistic infertility treatment option for certain couples, but also provides a unique model to investigate the endocrinology of early human pregnancy.

That pregnancy can be maintained by the administration of exogenous oestradiol and progesterone would suggest that of the various ovarian hormones,

Estimated timing of natural events in vivo

Cycle day	12	13	14	15	16	17	18	19	20	21	22	23	24	25
Event	Start LH surge	Start P$_4$	Fertilization / Ovulation	2-cell	4-cell	8-cell / 16-cell	Morula / Unhatched blastocyst	Hatched blastocyst		Commencement of implantation				

Relative timing of pregnancies reported to date

Source	Timeline events	Embryo ahead of uterus by (hours)	Embryo behind uterus by (hours)	Number of pregnancies reported
Monash IVF programme	P$_4$ (day 15); 2-cell, 3-cell; 2 × 4-cell, 1 × 6-cell, 3 × 8-cell	36–18		7
Feichtinger and Kemeter (1985)	P$_4$ (day 13); Fertilization	18		1
Navot et al. (1986)	P$_4$ (day 15); 4-6-cell (day 18), 4-6-cell (day 19)		4–28	2
Rosenwaks (1987)	P$_4$ (day 16); Transfers		0–48 (?)	8
Serhal and Craft (1987)	P$_4$ (day 14); Fertilization (day 15)		12	7
Asch et al. (1987)	P$_4$ (day 14); Fertilization	18		5

these steroids alone can provide the necessary endocrine environment for implantation and embryonic development. During early gestation in normal women the major progesterone source is the corpus luteum, and the importance of this structure in the maintenance of pregnancy was elegantly demonstrated in luteectomized rabbits using porcine corpus luteum extracts (Allan and Corner 1930). Csapo and co-workers confirmed these findings in women, showing that the effects of luteectomy, which results in abortion in early pregnancy, can be overcome by exogenous progesterone (Csapo et al. 1973). As pregnancy advances, the relative contribution of the corpus luteum to circulating progesterone concentrations falls, and the output of progesterone from the trophoblast increases. The luteo-placental shift in progesterone production is usually complete about 49 days after the last menstrual period in the human, following which the trophoblast alone is competent to provide the endocrine requirements to maintain pregnancy until term (Csapo and Pulkkinen 1978).

It would, therefore, be anticipated that to maintain pregnancy in agonadal women, exogenous steroid replacement should only be required for about 5 weeks following embryo transfer. In practice, we have continued steroid administration for 10 weeks post-transfer (range 5–17). Attempts at steroid withdrawal 6–8 weeks after transfer have caused significant reductions in circulating progesterone concentrations in particular, and although this may not necessarily result in abortion, it has been considered appropriate to err on the side of caution, and to try steroid withdrawal again at a later date.

11.7.2 Inhibin

Pregnancy in agonadal women permits assessment of the endocrine output of the human conceptus without interference from confounding ovarian factors. One such factor is inhibin.

The existence of a seminal pituitary-inhibiting agent was first postulated following the observation of castration-induced pituitary-cell hyperplasia (Mottram and Cramer 1923), and the name "inhibin" was suggested 9 years later to describe an active principle from bovine testes that could inhibit the appearance

---

Fig. 11.3. Summary of data on implantation in women receiving steroid replacement therapy to show variations in uterine–embryonic synchrony. The relative timing of embryonic stage of development and the elapsed time since the uterus first sees progesterone is given for 29 pregnancies (IVF and GIFT) in women without ovarian function. In some cases it is not possible to deduce the exact timing from the information in the literature. In the pregnancies achieved by Serhal and Craft (1987) and Asch et al. (1987) luteal progesterone commenced over a range of days; however, fertilization always occurred within a fixed time relationship of the commencement of progesterone. The data presented indicate that a window of uterine receptivity may extend for 36 hours before until 48 hours after the normal time that implantation occurs, i.e. from the start of day 19 until the end of day 23 of the standardized 28-day cycle. Further data are required to confirm and extend these observations.

These results show that successful pregnancies have been achieved with the embryo anything from 36 hours in front to 48 hours behind the uterus in terms of relative synchrony. It is possible that this 3-day "window" may be broadened further as more donor oocyte programmes are established. A second possibility is that future research will provide more detailed information on the uterine factors that govern the receptivity "window", thus allowing its manipulation and extension.

of these pituitary "castration cells" (McCullagh 1932). The structure of this putative inhibitor of pituitary follicle stimulating hormone (FSH) release has recently been described: isolation, cloning, and sequencing of the inhibin molecule has revealed that it comprises two peptide chains, A and B, linked by disulphide bridges (see McLachlan et al. 1987a for review).

Although inhibin has been demonstrated as a circulating peptide hormone with inhibitory effects on pituitary FSH release, the discovery of homology between inhibin, transforming Growth-Factor-β (Derynck et al. 1985), and Mullerian Inhibitory Substance (Cate et al. 1986), has suggested the possibility of additional regulatory roles for this compound.

Inhibin has been measured in the maternal circulation within 3 weeks of embryo transfer in three agonadal women, pregnant following oocyte donation (McLachlan et al. 1987b). Inhibin concentrations rose throughout pregnancy, and in two women circulating FSH concentrations were suppressed to within normal limits in the week after embryo transfer. These data confirm the ability of the early human conceptus to synthesize inhibin, and subsequent studies have demonstrated the presence of inhibin RNA in the bovine fetal gonad (Hodgson et al. 1987). An additional homology exists between transforming Growth-Factor-β and a pattern-controlling gene in *Drosophila* (Padgett et al. 1987). Coupled with the measurement of inhibin in early human pregnancy it is tempting to speculate a role for inhibin, or a structurally closely related compound, in the regulation of early embryonic development.

11.7.3 Delivery

Six agonadal woman at Monash have now been delivered of seven healthy babies (one twin pregnancy). In each case, elective Caesarian section was performed.

On subjective assessment, the term cervix remained unripe, although none of the women was allowed to proceed to spontaneous labour. A failure of cervical effacement and dilation could result from deficient relaxin production, for it is generally accepted that relaxin is produced by the corpus luteum (O'Byrne et al. 1978; Szalachter et al. 1980), although a decidual source has been reported (Bigazzi et al. 1983). The role of relaxin in women without ovarian function remains unclear, and further studies are therefore required to assess relaxin production in agonadal women conceiving on the donor oocyte programme.

11.8 Legal Aspects

Ethical and legal problems may be associated with the donor oocyte programme, and public debate and limited legislation are needed to safeguard its work. This has already been achieved in the State of Victoria, Australia. The Infertility (Medical Procedures) Act passed in 1984 supported the concept of oocyte donation. This Act stipulated that no payment be made to a woman for the donation of her oocytes. It also stated that non-identifying information regarding the oocyte donor should be made available to the recipient, who in turn should be offered non-identifying information regarding the recipient. This Act was further supported by the Status of Children (Amendment) Act (1984) which stated that the recipient woman "shall be presumed, for all purposes, to have become pregnant as a result of the fertilization of an ovum produced by her and to be the mother of any child born as a result of the pregnancy". This statute proclaims that the recipient of a donor oocyte pregnancy is the legal mother, and the oocyte donor has no legal right or responsibilities towards the child.

References

Allan WM, Corner GN (1930) Physiology of corpus luteum. VII. Maintenance of pregnancy in rabbit after very early castration, by corpus luteum extracts. Proc Soc Exp Biol Med 27:403–405

Asch R, Balmaceda J, Ord T et al. (1987) Oocyte donation and gamete intrafallopian transfer as treatment for premature ovarian failure. Lancet I:687–688

Bigazzi M, Nardig E, Petrucci F et al. (1983) Synthesis of relaxin by human decidua. In: Bigazzi M, Greenwood FC, Gasparri F (eds) Biology of Relaxin and its Role in the Human. Excerpta Medica, Amsterdam, pp 206–212

Bustillo M, Buster J, Cowen S (1984) Delivery of a healthy infant following non-surgical ovum transfer. JAMA 251:889

Cate RL, Mattaliano RJ, Hessian C et al. (1986) Isolation of the bovine and human genes for Mullerian inhibiting substance and expression of the human gene in animals. Cell 45:685–698

Csapo AI, Pulkkinen MO (1978) Indispensability of the human corpus luteum in the maintenance of early pregnancy. Luteo-placental shift in progesterone source. Obstet Gynecol Survey 33:69–81

Csapo AI, Pulkkinen MO, Wiest NG (1973) Effects of luteectomy and progesterone replacement therapy in early pregnancy patients. Am J Obstet Gynecol 115:759–765

Derynck R, Jarrett JA, Chen EY et al. (1985) Human transforming growth factor-β complementary DNA sequence and expression in normal and transformed cells. Nature 316:701–705

Devroey P, Smitz J, Wisanto A et al. (1987) Primary ovarian failure: embryo donation after substitution therapy. 5th world congress on IVF and ET. Norfolk, Virginia, 5–10 April (Abstract No OC–427)

Fawcett DW, Wislocki GB, Waldo CM (1947) The development of mouse ova in the anterior chamber of the eye and in the abdominal cavity. Am J Anat 81:413–443

Feichtinger W, Kemeter P (1985) Pregnancy after total ovariectomy achieved by ovum donation. Lancet II:722–723

Hodgson YM, Averill S, Torney A, de Kretser DM (1987) A fetal source of inhibin demonstrated by in situ hybridisation. Society for the study of fertility, York (abstract 41)

Kirby DRS (1963) The development of mouse blastocysts transplanted to the scrotal and cryptorchid testis. J Anat 97:119–130

Leeton J, Harman J (1986). Attitudes towards egg donation of thirty-four infertile women who donated during their in vitro fertilization treatment. J In Vitro Fertil Embryo Transfer 6:374–378

Leeton J, Harman J (1987) The donation of oocytes to known recipients. Aust NZ J Obstet Gynaecol 27:248–250

Leeton J, Trounson A, Jessup D, Wood C (1982) The technique for human embryo transfer. Fertil Steril 38:156–161

Leeton J, Chan C, Trounson A, Harman J (1986a) Pregnancy established in an infertile patient after transfer of an embryo fertilized in vitro where the oocyte was donated by the sister of the recipient. J In Vitro Fertil Embryo Transfer 6:379–382

Leeton J, Caro C, Howlett D, Harman J (1986b). The search for donor eggs: a problem of supply and demand. J Clin Reprod Fertil 4:337–340

Lenz S (1984) Ultrasonic guided aspiration of human oocytes. Ultrasound Med Biol 10:625–628

Lenz S, Leeton J, Renou P (1987) Transvaginal recovery of oocytes for in vitro fertilization using vaginal ultrasound. J In Vitro Fertil Embryo Transfer 4:51–55

Lutjen P, Trounson A, Leeton J, Findlay J, Wood C, Renou P (1984) The establishment and maintenance of pregnancy using in vitro fertilization and embryo donation in a patient with primary ovarian failure. Nature 307:174–175

Lutjen PJ, Findlay JK, Trounson AO, Leeton JF, Chan LK (1986) Effect on plasma gonadotropins of cyclic steroid replacement in women with premature ovarian failure. J Clin Endocrinol Metab 62:419–423

Mahadevan M, Trounson A, Leeton J (1983). Successful use of human semen cryobanking for in vitro fertilization. Fertil Steril 40:340–343

McLachlan RI, Robertson DM, de Kretser DM, Burger HG (1987a) Inhibin – a non-steroidal regulator of pituitary follicle stimulating hormone. Clin Endocrinol Metab 1:89–112

McLachlan RI, Healy DL, Lutjen PJ, Findlay JK, de Kretser DM, Burger HG (1987b) The maternal ovary is not the source of circulating inhibin levels during human pregnancy. Clin Endocrinol 27:663–668

McCullagh DR (1932) Dual endocrine control of the testes. Science 76:19–27

Muttram JC, Cramer W (1923) On the general effects of exposure to radium on metabolism and tumour growth in the rat and the special effects on testis and pituitary. QJ Exp Physiol 13:209–226

Murphy CR, Rogers PAW, Leeton J, Hosie M, Beaton L, Macpherson A (1987) Surface ultrastructure of uterine epithelial cells in women with premature ovarian failure following steroid hormone replacement. Acta Anat 130:348–350

Navot D, Lanfer N, Kopolovic J et al. (1986) Artificially induced endometrial cycles and establishment of pregnancies in the absence of ovaries. N Engl J Med 314:806–811

Noyes RW, Dickman Z (1960) Relationship of ovular age to endometrial development. J Reprod Fertil 1:186–196

Noyes RW, Hertig AT, Rock J (1950) Dating the endometrial biopsy. Fertil Steril 1:3–25

O'Byrne EM, Flitcraft JF, Sawyer WR, Hochman J, Weiss G, Steinetz BG (1978) Relaxin bioactivity and immunoactivity in human corpora lutea. Endocrinology 102:1641–1644

Padgett RW, Johnston D St, Gelbart WM (1987) A transcript from a drosophilia pattern gene predicts a protein homologous to the transforming growth factor-β family. Nature 325:81–84

Psychoyos A, Casimiri V (1981) Uterine blastotoxic factors. In: Glasser SR, Bullock DW (eds) Cellular and molecular aspects of implantation. Plenum Press, New York, pp 327–334

Rogers PAW, Milne B, Trounson AO (1986) A model to show uterine receptivity and embryo viability following ovarian stimulation for in vitro fertilization. J In Vitro Fertil Embryo Transfer 3:93–98

Rogers PAW, Macpherson A, Beaton L (1988) Embryo implantation in the anterior chamber of the eye: effects on uterine allografts and the microvasculature. Ann NY Acad Sci (in Press)

Rosenwaks Z, Veeck LL, Hurg-Ching L (1986) Pregnancy following transfer of in vitro fertilized donated oocytes. Fertil Steril 45:417–420

Serhal P, Craft I (1987) Simplified treatment for ovum donation. Lancet I:687–688

Szalachter N, O'Bryne E, Goldsmith L et al. (1980) Myometrial inhibiting activity of relaxin-containing extracts of human corpora lutea of pregnancy. Am J Obstet Gynecol 136:584–589

Templeton A, Van Look P, Lumsden M et al. (1984) The recovery of pre-ovulatory oocytes using a fixed schedule of ovulation induction and follicle aspiration. Br J Obstet Gynaecol 91:148–154

Trounson A, Leeton J, Besanko M, Wood C, Conti A (1983) Pregnancy established in an infertile patient after transfer of a donated embryo fertilized in vitro. Br Med J 286:835–838

Walters DE, Edwards RG, Meistrich ML (1985) A statistical evaluation of implantation after replacing one or more human embryos. J Reprod Fertil 74:557–563

12 Infertility Counselling

Louise Bowen and Kay Oke

12.1 Introduction

Most people consider fertility is something to be controlled and that infertility affects "other people". The thousands of couples on in vitro fertilization (IVF) programmes reflect the reality that infertility affects one in ten couples trying to achieve a pregnancy.

A diagnosis of infertility is profoundly distressing and represents a major life crisis (Pfeffer and Woollett 1983). It is often easier to focus attention on new technological opportunities for reproduction than to acknowledge how much infertility hurts emotionally. Many infertility centres consider emotional well-being an integral part of infertility treatment and have, accordingly, appointed counsellors to their programmes.

12.2 Why Would Anyone Seek or Need Specialised Infertility Counselling?

All staff working in infertility centres need to recognize the emotional reaction engendered by a diagnosis of infertility and know that not all people will react in the same way to this diagnosis. In most cases the sorts of reactions shown by people can be dealt with and "normalized" by the medical and nursing staff involved with each couple. These staff are generally able to distinguish between couples who are coping with their anxieties and those who need more specialized counselling services.

Common reactions to infertility have been likened to those associated with grief (Eck Menning 1977). These include initial shock and disbelief coupled with frustration and anger. Depression and feelings of overwhelming sadness are common, as are feelings of guilt, particularly in relation to past activities. A sense of shame, loneliness and isolation can be long lasting.

Dealing with these reactions can lead to problems interacting with friends and relatives. Marital discord may increase and can commonly be accompanied by sexual problems (Shapiro 1982; Elstein 1975). Social situations involving children are often settings where emotional reactions to infertility are strongly felt and noticed by others. Much understanding is expected, but not always obtained, from family and friends of the pain expressed by infertile couples.

Most couples report strong emotional reactions at particular times during their infertility tests and treatment. Many will deal with those feelings, appropriately, within their marriage, family or friendship circle. Others will need more specialized help to acknowledge and deal appropriately with their feelings. Such help can enable couples to deal constructively with their existing relationships and to remain open to the development of new ones.

The decision to seek counselling outside their own close networks can be a difficult one for couples who have never experienced or anticipated needing such help with their lives. When people are anxious it is important to deal sensitively with the sort of reactions common to those facing infertility. Counselling referrals should be made such that people feel they will be helped by discussion rather than feeling they are being punished for an inability to cope effectively at some point.

12.3   Is Counselling Synonymous with "Assessment"?

Many couples seeking, or referred for, infertility counselling assume they are to be "assessed" as to their suitability for parenthood. This may reflect the fact that many infertile couples explore adoption as a possibility and have assumptions about the adoption process being such an assessment.

The infertility counsellor's role is to help couples determine their own needs and make decisions appropriate to them. Counselling can help in the clarification and acknowledgement of problem areas, enabling couples to recognize the source and nature of pressures on them. The counsellor will also work with programme staff to ensure they are aware of couples needing additional attention whilst undergoing treatment.

Such an assessment is *not* synonymous with the notion of the counsellor accepting or rejecting a couple's suitability to proceed with treatment. Rather, this reflects a programme's attempt to ensure positive participation by acknowledging the emotional needs of its clients. Studies done on IVF couples indicate that as a group they have no major psychological dysfunction which would warrant any "exclusion" assessment (Greenfeld and Haseltine 1986).

12.4   Who Does the Counselling?

All medical and nursing staff who have ongoing contact with clients will have a counselling component in their work. For more specialized and intensive counselling it is most common for a social worker or psychologist to be appointed.

Practices vary greatly between programmes in the implementation of counselling services. Some programmes routinely administer psychological tests to help determine which couples may need additional psychological intervention or support (Greenfeld et al. 1984). Some programmes make counselling, either on an individual or group basis, an integral part of a couple's initiation and orientation, whilst others provide counselling on an as-needed basis. There has to date been no comparison between programmes to determine which system best meets the needs of its clients or, indeed, to determine if there is any way of providing a standardized, optimum service.

12.5   What Are Common Expressions Indicating Consideration of a Counselling Referral?

The following statements and questions are both commonly expressed and normal:

"I feel as though I'm going mad."

"No one understands what I'm going through; they try but they don't know."

"People keep telling me to relax or take a holiday. If I was more relaxed would I be more likely to get pregnant?"

"How can I stop feeling angry and cheated when friends get pregnant?"

"How can I help my partner cope better?"

"Our sex life has deteriorated – is this normal?"

"How do other people manage?"

Staff hearing such questions need to be receptive to their expression, neither dismissing them nor persnally taking on the helpless feelings often associated with them. Couples may seek specific exercises or strategies for dealing with these reactions such as yoga or relaxation therapy. Whilst such strategies can be enormously beneficial it is important for couples to also recognize and acknowledge the basis for their feelings. Exercise or relaxation-based strategies may not help if the reasons for these feelings remain unrecognized. A counsellor can help by planning together with a couple which avenues are most appropriate to their needs at a particular time.

Some see referral to a counsellor as indicating that their infertility is thought to be psychogenic. Particularly for those couples with a diagnosis of idiopathic infertility, there is the fear that the inability to conceive is caused by a subconscious desire not to have children. Psychogenic causes for infertility remain an area of conjecture with little data available. There is no current scientific evidence to indicate that infertility is of psychogenic origin in more than a very small number of cases (Christie 1980). Comments such as "just relax and you'll get pregnant" cause additional anxieties, doubts and pressures. A more positive and productive emphasis is to encourage relaxation with the aim of enhancing a couple's ability to deal with infertility and life in general (Eck Menning 1980).

12.6 When Is Infertility Counselling Appropriate?

IVF programmes should ensure that the emotional needs of their clients are determined individually, bearing in mind that each partner, too, will have individual needs. Thus the time when counselling is most appropriate will vary. Services should be easily accessible to people throughout their infertility treatment, from initial investigations to the ending of all active treatment.

It is possible to identify some obvious points of stress associated with IVF programmes. At these times, unexpected and often intense reactions can compound the many and complex reactions to the infertility itself. There are also times when particular decisions about treatment options must be made, decisions which are most appropriately dealt with in a counselling setting.

12.6.1 Initial Diagnosis of Infertility

This can be a time of confusion about the implications of a diagnosis, often leading to an exploration of both medical options and alternatives such as adoption or foster care. The counsellor needs to have a good working knowledge of the medical procedures and community resources which couples may wish to explore. The counsellor is then in a position to help clarify a couple's understanding of their problem and discuss the implications of each option to be considered.

12.6.2 Waiting List

Placement on an IVF waiting list can emphasize that there really *is* a problem. Couples may experience ambivalence about being on a list, particularly if they are still hoping for a natural conception. Waiting lists for programmes can be up to two years long. Whilst some people report that this time passes quickly, others need help to cope with the frustration associated with feeling that they are just "marking time".

12.6.3 First Treatment Cycle

This is often reported as the most emotionally demanding cycle, combining a mixture of high hopes and apprehension about procedures. Couples undergoing IVF usually consider themselves well able to cope with disappointments, feeling very experienced at this. Some report surprise at the intensity of their emotional reactions during this first cycle, particularly if it is unsuccessful.

12.6.4 Pregnancy Test

This formally marks the end of a treatment cycle, in most cases marking an unsuccessful attempt. The time preceding this test is reported as perhaps the most anxiety provoking and stressful time in a cycle. Despite knowing the statistical chances of pregnancy, some people are surprised that although the cycle went smoothly, a pregnancy was not achieved. Medical explanations are often sought for this; explanations which are usually unable to be given definitively. Some couples may need help to adjust to the idea that medical technology does not yet have all the answers in this area.

12.6.5 Timing of Next Attempt

At some point couples have to determine the number and timing of IVF cycles, particularly if the programme imposes no set limits. Some may need encouragement to take extended breaks between cycles or even to discontinue treatment. The safe environment of a counselling setting can be an appropriate place for couples to discuss their options and make plans to suit their particular needs.

12.6.6. Deciding to Finish IVF Treatment

This can represent a dilemma for some couples. It is difficult to think clearly about child-free lifestyle whilst undergoing treatment with obvious hopes for success. On the other hand it can be difficult to stop all active treatment until thoughts about lifestyle options can be faced with some equanimity. Reaching the point where the decision to stop has to be faced can be traumatic for some couples. Emotional reactions can be very mixed, involving both anguish and a sense of relief, and the decision can be something over which couples struggle.

It will not always be the case that each partner will simultaneously feel ready to stop treatment. The counsellor can help people review their experiences of infertility testing and treatment, perhaps helping each to understand why their partner is at a different stage. Acknowledging the feelings of each partner can enable couples to start working on their resolution to stop treatment and the implications of this on their lives together. In our experience it can be helpful for couples to use counselling sessions to work up to their final treatment rather than "after the event" counselling, particularly if uncertainty about stopping is an issue for one or both partners.

Sometimes the decision to stop treatment is made by achieving a pregnancy, an event which can be greeted with a mixture of joy and anxiety. Whilst most couples are able to deal with pregnancy-related anxieties within their own support networks, some may seek counselling to talk through fears and fantasies.

12.7 Should Counselling Be Mandatory for All Couples Seeking IVF?

The information-giving and decision-making aspects of counselling should be made available as a matter of routine, to all couples. This, however, must be distinguished from any therapeutic counselling which, by its very nature, cannot be compulsorily introduced.

12.8   Are There Particular Treatment Options Necessitating Prior Counselling?

For most couples, the decision to proceed to IVF treatment using their own gametes poses no particular moral, ethical or social difficulties. Family and friends usually know about and support participation in a treatment programme. This means that decisions about treatment options can often be discussed and determined using the couple's usual support network.

Some couples, however, have to consider the use of donor gametes from known or anonymous donors, donor embryos or surrogacy arrangements. These choices have particular emotional, social, legal and ethical implications which are important to confront prior to treatment decisions being made.

Many of these couples choose, at least initially, to consider these treatment options in secrecy, isolated from their most obvious support network of family and friends. It is quite common for couples using donor gametes not to have discussed their alternatives and feelings in great depth with each other by the time treatment options are put to them.

12.9   What Are the Particular Issues a Counsellor Would Discuss with Couples Contemplating the Use of Donor Gametes?

A counsellor will acknowledge issues, discuss implications and sometimes challenge assumptions couples make about the use of donor gametes. Areas to be covered will include:

1. *Secrecy*. There are many viewpoints about whether or not to tell a child about its origins when using donor gametes. The points for and against telling a child, family and friends need to be explored so couples make their own decisions in the most informed way. It is not always possible to think ahead to expected reactions should a pregnancy occur and the counsellor should be available throughout the treatment process and beyond. This is particularly relevant for couples who have decided from the outset to maintain the secrecy of their treatment choices.

2. *Genetic relationships*. Parenting a child who is genetically unrelated to one or both parents can give rise to many concerns. Questions about the donor need to be addressed openly with each couple. This allows any fears or fantasies about the donor to be dealt with in a safe and supportive environment.

3. *Self-esteem*. This can be damaged during infertility testing and treatment. The birth of a child from donor gametes can exacerbate these feelings rather than resolve them. If couples are well-prepared for possible reactions they are generally better able to recognise and deal with these reactions later on.

4. *Legal situation*. The legal implications of using donor gametes varies between countries and states. Couples need to understand their legal status as

parents and any possible legal complications as a result of their use of donor gametes. In Victoria, the Register of Donor Births needs very careful explanation particularly in relation to long-term confidentiality.

5. *Outcomes*. Many wish to know how others have handled being on donor programmes and ask about long-term outcomes. Some may wish to meet other couples, perhaps in a group setting to discuss attitudes, feelings, fears, with people who have previously used donor gametes. To date there have been few long-term follow up studies of donor programmes (Clayton and Kovacs 1982).

The issues raised by the use of donor gametes are often difficult for couples to discuss openly together. Some fear that such discussion may be painful, particularly to the infertile partner and that this could be destructive to their relationship. When communication is not open on this issue it often reflects the false hope that any problems will either not arise or will go away in time. Providing a safe and accepting environment to explore difficult areas encourages couples making such choices to feel that discussion is appropriate, healthy and comforting.

12.10   What Is the Counselling Role of Support Groups?

Many couples consider that only another infertile person can really understand what pain they are suffering; that it is obvious that fertile friends and family can only help to a limited extent. These couples may not consider they need professional help but wish to talk over their experiences with another infertile person. Support groups offer a number of services for couples on IVF programmes. These range from telephone counselling and referral services, group meetings and information sessions to political activities and fundraising events. Programme counsellors can work closely with support groups to facilitate contact between infertile couples and to represent client interests at the programme level.

References and Further Reading

Christie GL (1980) Psychological and social management. In: Pepperell R, Hudson B, Wood C (eds) The infertile couple. Churchill Livingstone, Edinburgh
Clayton C, Kovacs G (1982) AID offspring. Initial follow-up of 50 couples. Med J Aust 1:338
Eck Menning B (1977) Infertility – a guide for the childless couple. Prentice Hall, Englewood Cliffs
Eck Menning B (1980) The emotional needs of infertile couples. Fertil Steril 34:313
Elstein M (1975) Effect of infertility on psychosexual function. Br Med J iii:296
Freeman EW, Garcia CR, Rickels K (1983) Behavioural and emotional factors: comparisons of anovulatory infertile women with fertile and other infertile women. Fertil Steril 40:195
Friedman R, Gradstein B (1982) Surviving pregnancy loss. Little, Brown, Boston
Greenfeld D, Haseltine F (1986) Candidate selection and psychosocial consideration of in-vitro fertilisation procedures. Clin Obstet Gynaecol 29:119–126
Greenfeld D, Mazure C, Haseltine F, Decherney A (1984) The role of the social worker in the in-vitro fertilisation program. Soc Work Health Care 10:71–79

Keye WJ Jr (1986) The emotional aspects of infertility: a neglected problem. FSA Conference, Adelaide 1986

Kubler Ross E (1970) On death and dying. Tavistock, London

Leeton J, Backwell J (1982) A preliminary psycho-social follow-up of parents and their children conceived through artificial insemination by donor (AID). Clin Reprod Fertil (1982) 1:307–310

Noyes RW, Charnick EM (1964) Literature on psychology and infertility – a critical analysis. Fertil Steril 15:543

Pfeffer N, Woollett A (1983) The experience of infertility. Virago, London

Shapiro CH (1982) The impact of infertility on the marital relationship. Social Casework. 63:387–393

Snowden R, Snowden E (1984) The gift of a child. George Allen and Unwin, London

Stanway A (1980) Why us? Granada Publishing, London

Subject Index